STUDY SKILLS FOR PARAMEDICS

AND OTHER HEALTHCARE PROFESSIONALS

FIRST EDITION

STUDY SKILLS FOR PARAMEDICS

AND OTHER HEALTHCARE PROFESSIONALS

HELEN COBB
Paramedicine Lecturer, Edith Murphy House
De Montford University
The Gateway, Leicester, Leicestershire
United Kingdom

EMILY FORSTER
Lecturer in Learning, De Montford University
The Gateway, Leicester, Leicestershire
United Kingdom

ELSEVIER   For additional online content visit ExpertConsult.com

---

Notices

Practitioners and researchers must always rely on their own experience and knowledge in evaluating and using any information, methods, compounds or experiments described herein. Because of rapid advances in the medical sciences in particular, independent verification of diagnoses and drug dosages should be made. To the fullest extent of the law, no responsibility is assumed by Elsevier, authors, editors or contributors for any injury and/or damage to persons or property as a matter of product liability, negligence or otherwise, or from any use or operation of any methods, products, instructions or ideas contained in the material herein.

ISBN: 978-0-7020-8305-1

Content Strategist: Poppy Garraway
Content Development Specialist: Andrae Akeh
Publishing Services Manager: Shereen Jameel
Project Manager: Aparna Venkatachalam
Design Direction: Ryan Cook
Illustration Manager: Anitha Rajarathnam

Printed in India

Last digit is the print number: 9 8 7 6 5 4

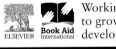

Working together
to grow libraries in
developing countries

www.elsevier.com • www.bookaid.org

CONTENTS

STUDY SKILLS FOR PARAMEDICS

AND OTHER HEALTHCARE PROFESSIONALS

INTRODUCTION

THIS CHAPTER WILL:

- Introduce the book to you, including a brief discussion around the different study levels.
- Explain how university education works and how it is developing, as well as different teaching approaches, including one called the flipped classroom approach, and what will be expected of you as students.
- Recognize the practical nature of paramedics and other allied healthcare practitioners and attempt to reassure you as a student that a step-by-step, gradual approach will get you to where you want to be: out working in the ambulance service or in a healthcare setting.
- Provide a basic explanation of the general set-up of the book to make it easier to read and get through.
- Include a chat about different learning needs (for example, dyslexia) and also address any worries you might have as a student who is new to higher education or as a student who feels he or she is not coping with the study skills element of his or her course.

STOP—BREATHE—CONTINUE

So What Is This Book About?

Ultimately, as students, you are actually going to have to do some academic work at some point, be it essays, exams, role play, presentations…the list goes on and on. Granted, it might not be your favourite part of the course, but remember: if you want to pass, you are going to have to put the effort in (Fig. 1.1).

This book has been designed to assist you, the student, in passing your assignments; that is its only purpose! It has been deliberately designed to cut out the waffle and the 'nice to know' information and to actually tell you what you need to know.

As a paramedic, an allied health student or (let's be honest) a student in general, you probably have not got either the time or the inclination to read 10 books on how to write an essay or to trawl through pages and pages of information to work out how to formulate a title, so let's miss that out and get to the facts.

So How Does the Book Work?

Each chapter will focus on one area of assessment, so it will be easy for you to refer directly to the chapter you need. Then, there will be a couple of generic chapters that cover topics that will help you in the majority of assessments, for example, literature searches or references.

> There will also be tricks and tips boxes just like this one, which will include areas that we think are really important and will hopefully get you moving forward quickly.

Finally, there will be examples that will be related directly to healthcare. Hopefully this will help you to put what we are saying into action.

So Where Now?

First of all, don't worry, everyone in your group has probably come from a different background and has different strengths and weaknesses. (Yes, we said weaknesses, which is not a term used in higher education much; you might hear 'areas for improvement' instead!)

Someone, it might be you, could write an essay in 2 hours and get top marks (annoying for everyone else, but definitely good for the student involved); for others it might take 3 weeks. Then again, someone might be able to undertake an objective structured clinical examination, most commonly known as an OSCE (we will talk about OSCEs later, but they are

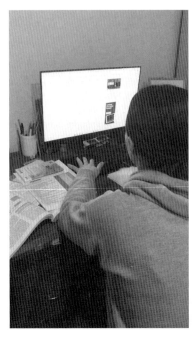

Fig. 1.1 Work, work, work.

basically medical scenarios, and you are marked against a marking sheet), without a care in the world, whereas others might be up for 2 days worrying about it (Fig. 1.2).

What we are trying to say is: don't worry! Everyone is different, and this book will help everyone get to grips with what needs to be done to pass.

University education probably works completely differently to what you are used to. There are different styles of teaching, and that really depends on the lecturer and the module you are taking. We know it doesn't help that lecturers are

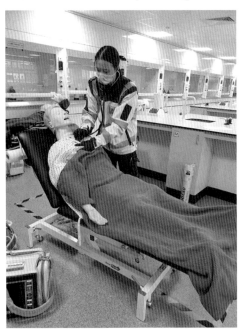

Fig. 1.2 Objective structured clinical examination (OSCE) practice.

all different if you like one set style, but at least you shouldn't get bored with all the variety. Some of the different kinds of teaching styles you could encounter might be:

- Lectures
- Seminars
- Workshops
- Simulations
- Webcasts

Often at universities nowadays you are given prelearning assignments before sessions and postlearning assignments after sessions. The first question we would ask is: why can't they teach me all I need to know in the lessons, so I don't have to do extra work at home? After all, I won't be taking my patients home when I'm trained, so why do I have to do the extra work outside of university when I'm in training?

The answer is a simple one: there is so much to learn that there is not enough time to teach you everything you need to know. Could you sit in 7 hours of lecture 5 days a week about human anatomy and all the complicated stuff that comes alongside, and actually take it all in? We know you couldn't.

Therefore, the university drive is on self-directed learning to enhance the teaching you get from your lecturers. Without this self-directed learning you may well struggle in your studies, irrespective of your course, so the first tip of the day is:

> Make sure you do the pre- and postlecture tasks. They are often designed to help with your final assessment.

Also, undertaking the pre- and poststudy is a necessity, because often universities use an approach called the 'flipped classroom' approach. This is where the basic reading comes before the session, and then the university session takes an in-depth look at the subject, so if you don't do the prelearning you will not understand the classroom lesson.

WHY THE BOOK?

This book is designed to help you get through the assessments you have probably been dreading (well, the first one anyway) and will enable you to progress through your course to become a paramedic or allied health professional. After all, the health professionals are very practical; we just need to get through the academic bits to be able to get the jobs!

When you are entering into a practical profession such as healthcare, some question why any academic work is needed. After all, if the job is by its nature practical, why be assessed on essays, or in fact any kind of written assignment?

Well, these trades are progressive, and it has been deemed by governing bodies such as the Health Care Professional Council, the College of Paramedics and the Nursing and Midwifery Council, alongside other healthcare regulatory bodies, that a higher standard of education is required to make the professions both effective and contemporary (this means modern or up-to-date; sorry if you know this already, but it is something I had not heard of before coming into higher education).

Every profession that is covered by the scope of this book is progressive, and more and more is being expected of the individuals that are choosing these professions. This, therefore, leads to a higher standard of education, which, in turn, requires more knowledge to be demonstrated by you the students, that is, more assignments.

Before you start worrying, the build-up within academia (yep, the university system) is gradual, and there are various elements associated with each academic level.

There are three academic levels that are taught during a degree:

- 1st year = level 4 (a certificate in higher education)
- 2nd year = level 5 (a diploma in higher education)
- 3rd year = level 6 (a full degree—either BSc or BA)

Later on in this book we will look at what will be expected of you at each level.

It is also important to remember that the mark needed to pass at university is generally a lot lower than in your previous places of study; often a pass benchmark is 40% (this is dependent, however, on the piece of work; for example, the benchmark for a paramedic pharmacy exam will be much higher because of the critical nature of what is being examined). Your final grading or degree classification is taken from your level 5 and 6 work, not your level 4 work, so consider level 4 as the 'getting it right' year!

Degree classifications are determined by your average percentage across year 2 and 3, so remember that you need to work hard on every assessed piece of work if you want to get a 1st-class degree. If you get 40% throughout, you should expect a 3rd-class degree. You will still gain registration, but it might affect you when trying to access courses further on in your career because some places want a 2:1 or a 1st-class degree (just like to get into university you need to get the right number of UCAS points). What we're trying to say is: don't coast—work hard.

DYSLEXIA AND SPECIFIC LEARNING DIFFICULTIES

This book has also been designed to ensure that it is practical and usable across all scopes of learning difficulty. According to Higher Education Statistics Agency (2020) data, in 2018/19 228, 345 of students enrolled in higher education in the United Kingdom had a declared disability, including specific learning difficulties such as dyslexia.

There are lots of paramedics and healthcare professionals with specific learning difficulties, and this shouldn't slow down your career. There is so much support available at all universities now that it won't slow anyone down.

If you think you have a learning difficulty, ask for an assessment early, and then you will have support throughout your time at university. However, even if you don't have a diagnosis of a learning difficulty, if you are struggling there is always help available. A good point of contact is the library; often, they offer drop-in sessions. There should be someone who is responsible for teaching study skills (this is sometimes called learning development) who you can see.

> Don't struggle in silence.

REFERENCES

HESA. (2020). Figure 4—HE student enrolments by personal characteristics 2014/15 to 2018/19. Available at: https://www.hesa.ac.uk/data-and-analysis/sb252/figure-4. Accessed on 31/07/2020.

HESA. (2021). Higher Education Student Statistics: UK, 2019/20 - Student numbers and characteristics. Available at: https://www.hesa.ac.uk/news/27-01-2021/sb258-higher-education-student-statistics/numbers. Accessed on 18/06/2021.

ACADEMIC WRITING

IN THIS CHAPTER:

- We start by looking at what makes writing academic and discuss the four main features: formal, evidence-based, cautious and critical writing.
- Next we look at writing at different levels and how the expectations will change as you progress through your degree.
- After that we discuss the writing process, with tips for success at different stages of writing.
- Then we tell you how to understand what you need to do and give some guidance on interpreting an assignment brief.
- Finally we finish with some tips on writing with clarity and how to avoid some of the most common errors we see in student essays.

Firstly, academic writing is new to the vast majority of level 4 students. All you need to know is it is a language, and once you have learnt it, it will be much easier for you.

UNDERSTANDING WHAT YOU NEED TO DO

Before you can write you need to understand what it is you need to do, and for this you will have an assignment brief.

For every assignment you do, you will be given an assignment brief telling you what you need to do. These briefs might be presented in different ways at different universities, such as on an A4 sheet, within a presentation or on a virtual learning site such as Moodle or Blackboard. It is important to stick to the brief and not go off on a tangent. The brief will include the learning outcomes of the assignment, and these are key to passing.

Make sure you understand the assignment brief: without understanding exactly what you have to do, what chance do you have of getting it correct?

Also, look at the marking criteria if they are provided (if not, then ask the tutor): then you will know what you need to do to get that elusive 1st class qualification. Once you have the criteria, make sure you study them and understand them.

WHAT MAKES WRITING ACADEMIC?

There are four features of academic writing:
- It is formal in style
- It is evidence based
- It is often cautious in tone
- It often includes critical analysis (depending on academic level)

Although this is true for all academic writing, different assignments have slightly different rules. Don't worry about that too much, though, because this book will help you make sense of the different types of assignments you need to write for university and what is expected of you.

Let's have a look at each feature a little more closely.

FORMALITY

The first and most obvious feature of academic writing is that it is formal in style. You obviously (I hope) wouldn't write an essay for university in the same style that you would use to write a text message to a friend or a post on social media—'LOL' in a formal assignment is just not setting the right tone—but there are some other features that you might not have considered.

Just because it is formal, that does not mean that you need to use fancy words and sound like you have swallowed a dictionary. You want to communicate your ideas as clearly as you can (a really important skill for any healthcare professional). Depending on what you are writing about you may need to use the correct medical vocabulary and technical terms, and this can make things complicated enough. The aim is to get your thinking down and make sure it is clear and well thought-out.

> Avoid using colloquialisms. These are phrases that can be used in everyday language, like 'at the end of the day' or 'I wasn't born yesterday'.

> Use the full version of the words rather than the abbreviated version:
> 'do not' rather than 'don't', 'defibrillator' rather than 'defib', 'technology' rather than 'tech'… you get the drift (that was a colloquialism, by the way).

> Do not use emotive language. Sometimes if you are discussing something you are passionate about, it can be difficult, but avoiding words such as 'tragic', 'dreadful' or 'horrific' can actually mean that your work is taken more seriously.

EVIDENCE-BASED WRITING

Another thing that makes academic writing different from other forms of writing is that everything you say needs to be supported by high-quality evidence (this is covered in more detail in the literature search chapter). This affects the way you approach a writing task because before you can start to write you need to do some research and get an idea of what the medical evidence says. When you write you need to include a reference to the evidence in the text. This is such a big part of academic writing (and one of the things that students most stress about when they start university) that we have included a whole chapter on referencing and using evidence, so try to relax.

The main thing you need to get to grips with is that whenever you are claiming that something is a fact you need to provide some evidence.

For example, rather than writing 'Diabetes is a very common medical condition', you would write 'An estimated 3.8 million people in the United Kingdom have been diagnosed with diabetes (Public Health England, 2018)' (Fig. 2.1).

What you are doing here is letting the evidence do the talking and proving that you know what you are talking about.

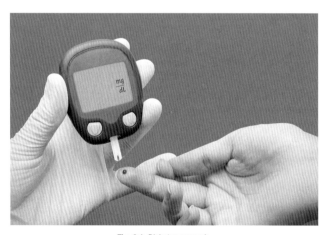

Fig. 2.1 Diabetes research.

CAUTIOUS TONE

When writing academically, often you need to write in the third person (this means not using I, my, me, etc.). For example, instead of writing 'I think that', you would say something like 'It is believed that'.

As a result of the focus on using evidence, academic writing tends to be cautious in style. As you have hopefully gathered, making bold claims that you can't support is out, as is putting your point of view across without any evidence (and that's high-quality evidence, not 'Bob's Really Useful Information website').

One approach people often use is letting the evidence do the talking for them, as you can see in the example below:

> **I think that** (diabetes is on the rise). **Evidence supports this** (The number of people with diabetes rose from 108 million in 1980 to 422 million in 2014 (WHO, 2018). **This proves that** (the number of cases of diabetes worldwide is increasing at a significant rate).

Make sure any key information you are putting in your assignment or paper is supported by evidence; otherwise, your work will not be taken seriously, and you will get a low grade or be unable to publish your paper.

GRADE DESCRIPTORS

Grade descriptors are basically a set of criteria (levels) that you have to work to, to get the grade you want to achieve in your assignments.

An organization called SEEC (2016) provided the guidance on what universities expect in the different years and levels of study. This guidance is used by most universities. Your university will have its own set of grade descriptors, and you should make yourself familiar with them. However, the descriptors often use quite complex language, so here is a simplified version:

Level 4/year 1
- Take responsibility for your own study
- Have a broad knowledge of the subject and be able to apply this
- Learn key academic skills such as referencing
- Write in an academic style using appropriate medical language
- Access sources and analyze them
- Learn core clinical skills
- Complete a placement where you are under supervision

Level 5/year 2
- Have a more detailed knowledge of your subject and be able to apply it to a wider range of contexts
- Understand the knowledge base of the subject and that more is known about some areas than others
- Feel secure in academic skills such as referencing
- Access a wider range of high-quality sources and critically evaluate them
- Be able to write in an academic style using appropriate medical vocabulary and show critical analysis
- Complete a placement with an increased level of independence and responsibility

Level 6/year 3
- Be able to find and critically review a wide range of sources
- Have a sound understanding of the knowledge base in your subject and be able to apply this to unfamiliar situations
- Feel secure in academic skills
- Be able to write in a polished academic style with strong critical analysis and synthesis of sources
- Complete a placement with increased levels of responsibility so that you are able to work autonomously by the end of your degree

CRITICAL ANALYSIS

One of the main things your lecturers will look for in a university-level assignment is critical analysis. If you look at any set of marking criteria, critical analysis will feature. As you progress through your degree, the level of critical analysis that you are expected to show increases.

One of the most common misunderstandings people have about critical analysis is that it means being negative, and that you need to look for faults in everything. However, critical analysis can be positive too. Obviously if there are flaws in any argument you can point them out, but you can also explain why something is relevant and useful, or why a piece of research supports your argument.

In the context of your paramedic or allied health qualification the main way you can demonstrate critical thinking is to show how you can apply your knowledge. You may be able to learn and remember a lot of facts and physical skills such at putting patients on a spinal board or inserting a cannula. This will serve you well when you graduate, but will not prove that you understand why you perform each action, and therefore you will not be able to pass your course and actually use your skills in the real world. Once you have graduated, it will make it much easier to justify skills or decisions in your head or to the Health and Care Professions Council if you understand why you perform each action and what the evidence is behind the skills (Fig. 2.2).

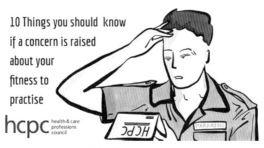

Fig. 2.2 HCPC fitness to practice.

At this point you may be thinking: this is all very well, but what does critical analysis look like in an assignment? The first thing that's looked at within the essay is whether you have presented a logical argument that leads to answering whatever question was set.

A really common point students receive within feedback is that their writing is too descriptive. This means something like:

> An extraction board is used to extricate patients with potential spinal injuries in cars, it used to be used to transport patients but now because of changes advised by … a scoop stretcher is mostly used instead because it is considered better for the patient.

It is not just enough to write what other people have said. You need to bring all this evidence together into one coherent answer:

It is believed that…this is supported by…however…states that this is not the case and…believes that, after consideration of the information, this paper deems that it is the case in the majority of situations that…

Your assignment should have an overall point and be structured in the best way to answer the question. This is sometimes referred to as the line of argument. This will make more sense if you have a look at the essay plan described later.

Remember that, in general, academic writing uses the third person. However, there are exceptions to this; for example, in reflective writing it is usual to write in the first person.

If you ask yourself critical questions, it is easier to formulate critical answers:
- What?
- Why?
- How?
- What if?

We have already identified that a common mistake is to presume that critical analysis has to be negative, and that you need to look for faults in everything. Do not forget that critical analysis can be positive too.

This model, which is used to generate critical thinking, was developed by John Hilsdon at Plymouth University (Hilsdon 2010). As you can see, there are three levels of critical questions, description, analysis and evaluation (Fig. 2.3).

Below are two more questions that you need to ask yourself:
- **How does this relate to my essay question?** It is important that you only include relevant information. If you go 'off topic' and effectively 'waffle' you will not be able to answer the question within the word count.
- **How could I use this information as a healthcare professional?** You need to actually link it to what you are studying and remember that if it is in an assignment it will actually be needed in your job in the future.

THE PROCESS OF WRITING AT UNIVERSITY

It is important to realize that writing is a process. A lot of students say that they cannot write, and initially it causes a lot of worry, but nobody produces a perfect piece of writing that gets across everything they want to say the first time.

Everything you will read for your assignment will have gone through many drafts. Don't compare your first draft to the finished product. This book has been edited a lot by a number of different people before it has reached you…trust us, we know!

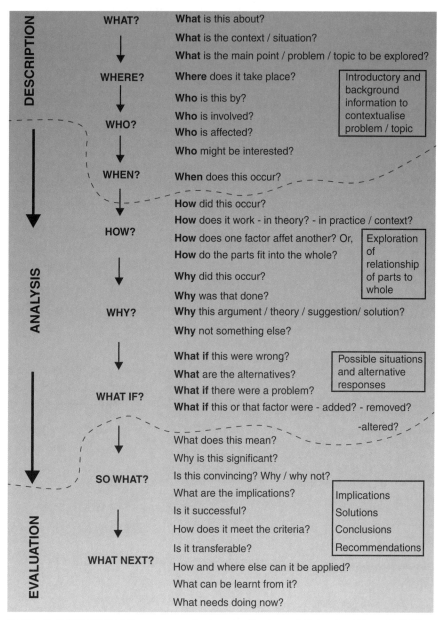

DESCRIPTION

WHAT?
What is this about?
What is the context / situation?
What is the main point / problem / topic to be explored?

WHERE?
Where does it take place?
Who is this by?
Who is involved?
WHO?
Who is affected?
Who might be interested?

WHEN?
When does this occur?

Introductory and background information to contextualise problem / topic

ANALYSIS

HOW?
How did this occur?
How does it work - in theory? - in practice / context?
How does one factor affet another? Or,
How do the parts fit into the whole?

Why did this occur?
Why was that done?
WHY?
Why this argument / theory / suggestion/ solution?
Why not something else?

Exploration of relationship of parts to whole

WHAT IF?
What if this were wrong?
What are the alternatives?
What if there were a problem?
What if this or that factor were - added? - removed?
-altered?

Possible situations and alternative responses

EVALUATION

SO WHAT?
What does this mean?
Why is this significant?
Is this convincing? Why / why not?
What are the implications?
Is it successful?
How does it meet the criteria?
Is it transferable?

WHAT NEXT?
How and where else can it be applied?
What can be learnt from it?
What needs doing now?

Implications
Solutions
Conclusions
Recommendations

Study guide 8: 'Critical Thinking' summary version, Learning Development, University of Plymouth (2009)

Fig. 2.3 Critical thinking.

WRITING AS A PROCESS

It is best to think of writing as a process. You are not going to get everything right the first time, nobody does. Part of the problem is that there are four different phases to writing, and a lot of people try to do all of them at the same time. If you are trying to think about what you want to say and worrying about your spelling at the same time, then you are going to stress yourself out unnecessarily. You will probably find yourself going backwards and forwards between these stages (Fig. 2.4).

Researching and planning. In this phase you are reading and making notes. You will be getting an idea of what your topic is and what you think about it. It is not possible to write a university-level assignment without doing any research or reading, as you need to know what the evidence says on this topic. Make sure that you keep track of everything you have read.

> Write down where you got EVERYTHING from: you will need this information later.

Writing. This is the bit where you actually do the writing. Try to focus on just getting the ideas down. You can always edit what you write later, but you can't edit a blank piece of paper! Once you have some key points down, it is much easier to get going. You can start by, just writing down what you plan to put in each section, and then build on it from there.

Editing. This is where you look at the draft and think about the structure, asking yourself whether what you are saying is presented in the most logical order. You might rearrange things, notice something you have missed out or realize that you

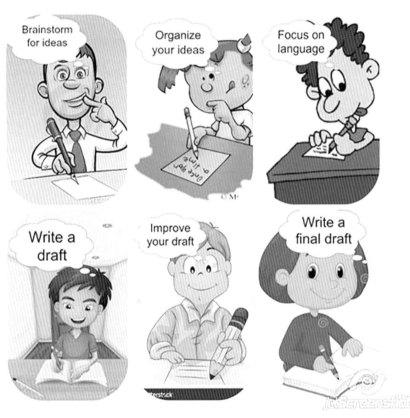

Fig. 2.4 Raise your essay score.

need to find more references. This is a really important part of the writing process, as you consider if what you have written actually makes sense and helps develop your critical analysis.

Questions to ask when editing:

- Does your introduction provide a good background to the assignment? (Remember: tell the reader what you are covering and why.)
- Is it clear what your argument or answer to the question is going to be?
- Are the sections in the most logical order?
- Do you present a consistent argument?
- Do you have enough evidence to support your ideas? (If in doubt, provide a reference; see the referencing chapter for more details.)
- Is it clear how the evidence supports your argument?
- Does the conclusion tell us exactly how you have answered the question?
- Does it leave the reader with a positive impression?
- Do all your sections link together?

Proofreading. This is the final stage in writing your assignment. People often confuse editing and proofreading, but editing focuses on more structural concerns (is everything in the right place, and have you answered the question?), whereas proofreading is just concerned with checking the spelling, punctuation, grammar and referencing.

Don't start proofreading until you have done the final edit because the text will change. Leave time for proofreading before your assignment needs to be handed in. You probably know how much this is an issue for you. See the advice on writing with clarity (this means writing without mistakes such as grammatical errors, using the right punctuation and bits like that) at the end of this chapter.

Most people have not done a lot of writing before they start at university. If this is the case, being asked to write a 2000-word report can send you into a blind panic. Don't worry, there are lots of things you can do to take away the fear of the blank page.

Some people have the opposite problem and end up writing way more than the word limit for the assignment and trying to cut bits out in a panic.

So what should you do if this happens?

GET WRITING

Many people find that when they sit down to write they have a voice in their head that tells them: 'Well this is a load of old rubbish. I don't know what I am doing, and what I have written is rubbish'.

If you feel like this, don't worry, you are not alone. You just have to wind it back a little and get something down on paper.

Here are some strategies that might help

Draw your essay (yes really!) or make a mind map

Here is a random example I have written for you (spelling mistakes and all; it really doesn't matter just get going)

Sometimes students struggle to get the information from their brains onto paper. Don't worry this is not uncommon I have this problem sometimes too. If you can't think of the right way of saying what you want to say, try the process below. That way you have four chances of getting it right:

- **Think it**—try and work it out in your head
- **Say it**—say what you want to write out loud (sometimes your university might have a software package such as Dragon that lets you dictate your work; ask the library if you are unsure)
- **Write it**—just write (or type out everything that comes out of your head)
- **Edit it**—once you have got it down, then you can spend time editing it; you might have surprised yourself

Sometimes you may simply need to talk to someone about it to start with if you are struggling or concerned. Often university libraries had drop-in sessions, and speaking to one of the advisors can be enough to get you going. If not, make an appointment with your tutor to talk you through the assignment. Make sure you start the assignment early; if not, your tutor might not have the capacity to see you.

WRITING WITH CLARITY

It will not come as a shock to anyone that to write a good assignment you need to have a high standard of spelling punctuation and grammar. Although this is not a book about grammar (you will be relieved to know), there are a few common mistakes that many people make. We will go over a few of them here so you know how to avoid them.

WRITING CLEAR SENTENCES

A sentence should make sense entirely on its own. All sentences must have two things: a subject and a finite verb. In the following examples, the subject is underlined, and the finite verb is in bold:

- An estimated 850,000 people in the United Kingdom **have** some form of dementia (Alzheimer's Society, 2017).
- Defibrillation **is** most effective if it is carried out within 3 to 5 minutes.

You don't always need to begin the sentence with the subject, but it is clearer if you do. Try to keep the finite verb close to the subject of the sentence because this makes it easier to follow.

Sentence Fragments

A sentence fragment is a sentence that does not make sense on its own because it lacks either a subject or a finite verb. For example:

Which means that urgent treatment is necessary.
There are two ways to fix a sentence fragment. One is to make it part of the previous sentence, separated by a comma: The patient was showing signs of sepsis, which means that urgent treatment is necessary.
The other is to change the sentence so it makes sense:
This means that urgent treatment is necessary.

Sentences That Are Too Long

One of the most common mistakes students make in their writing is to make their sentences go on for too long. This makes their writing very difficult to read (we have seen a whole page that was written as one long sentence). For example:

Paramedics often work with other healthcare professionals (HCPs) such as community nurses, general practitioners and midwives, this is so all the patients get the best possible standard of care from the right HCP. Paramedics carry out lots of duties such as vehicle checks, responding to 999 calls and safeguarding, this makes their job extremely varied.

As you can see, the student has joined the first two sentences together with a comma. If you have two parts of the sentence that would make sense on their own, then they should not be joined together with a comma. There are several things that you can do to fix this:
- Replace the full stop with a comma to make two sentences
- If the two sentences are continuing on in a similar point, you could join them together with a conjunction (for example, 'and' or 'but')
- You could replace the comma with either a semicolon or a colon
   In the example, a full stop would have been best.

APOSTROPHES (')

The apostrophe is without doubt the most abused and misused punctuation mark. People love to put apostrophes here, there and everywhere when they are not needed. There are two reasons to use an apostrophe:
- To indicate that somebody owns something. For example: 'the patient's belongings'. Here the apostrophe shows that the belongings are owned by the patient. If you had more than one patient, you would put the apostrophe after the s: 'the patients' belongings'.
- To indicate that a word has been shortened. For example, 'don't' is a contraction of 'do not'; 'won't' is a contraction of 'will not'. However, as we have already told you, it is not appropriate to use contractions in academic writing, you should write words out in full.
   Do not use an apostrophe to make a word plural (this means trying to say there are more than one). For example: 'the paramedic's all think assignments are hard work to write' is incorrect, and should be 'the paramedics all think assignments are hard work to write'.

EXCLAMATION MARKS

These should be used very sparingly. To be blunt, there are few examples of where it would be appropriate to use them in academic writing, so just do not use them.

COMMONLY CONFUSED WORDS

When you use spell check you might get the right spelling but the wrong word! These similar-sounding words are easily confused, so make sure you know the difference:
- There = in that place
   Their = belonging to them
   They're = they are
- Affect = to influence something
   Effect = something that was the result of something else.
   These are very similar. If you are not sure which one to use, try replacing it in the sentence with another verb. For example, 'this affects the patient's blood pressure' would also work as 'this lowers the patient's blood pressure', so 'affect' is the right one to use in this sentence.
- *Lose* = to misplace something—like the ambulance keys
   Loose = to become slack—you know, when your trousers are too big and fall down
- *Than* = is used when you are comparing something
   Then = is used to discuss time
- *Whose* = a possessive pronoun that means belonging to somebody (whose jumper is this?)
   Who's = a contraction of 'who is' (who's at the door?)

REFERENCES

Hilsdon, J. (2010). Critical thinking, University of Plymouth. Available at: https://www.plymouth.ac.uk/uploads/production/document/path/1/1710/Critical_Thinking.pdf. Accessed on 31/07/2020.

SEEC. (2016). Credit level descriptors for higher education [Online]. Available at: https://seec.org.uk/wp-content/uploads/2016/07/SEEC-descriptors-2016.pdf. Accessed on 11/06/2020.

WHO. (2018). Diabetes key facts. Available at: https://www.who.int/news-room/fact-sheets/detail/diabetes. Accessed on 12/05/2020.

NOTE-TAKING AND INFORMATION SOURCES

THIS CHAPTER DISCUSSES:

- Different reading strategies.
- Various note-taking strategies.

WHY DO WE NEED TO NOTE-TAKE AND FIND INFORMATION?

Because using evidence is so important in academic writing, you are going to need to do some reading. You will read to understand the evidence and learn more about a topic, and you will read to provide evidence for your assignments. Often these two things are linked.

READING STRATEGIES

There is so much reading to do at university; therefore, it is important to take a smart approach to reading. You don't have time to read every word of everything that you have on your reading list, nor do you need to. But you do need to have a good understanding of what you do read, otherwise you won't progress, and it will be a complete waste of your time. On top of that, your work won't make sense, which will lead to a low grade or failure—something we are trying to avoid.

Often there is a reading list given to you for each module. Start there when looking for books because more often than not lecturers make sure that the reading list covers what you need to know. Sometimes they use these sources to assist in lecture planning and content, so at least you know the information is correct!

What you need to do is simply read the most important and valuable parts of the text. You can skip the rest and come back to read it in more detail later if you need to.

Here are some strategies to help you.

HAVING QUESTIONS

Start by thinking about what you want to get out of reading this particular text. Do you want to use it in an assignment? Is there a particular aspect of the topic you need to find out about? If the text is not useful for your purpose, skip it and find something else to read.

It is always handy to write down what you are trying to find out. It will stop you forgetting when you go and get the fifth cuppa of the study session to put off reading for a little longer.

For example, if you are researching the treatment for a sprain, you might formulate the questions as 'is rest, ice compression and elevation considered best practice?' or 'what is the best pain relief for bone injuries?' (Fig. 3.1). If you get to a chapter in a book about the skeletal system, it might be worth a scan, but if it's about the circulatory system, don't bother looking!

(https://www.youtube.com/watch?v=10pwg9XQnS0)

A nice picture - who says you can't have medical images in a study skills book!

SKIMMING

When you skim-read the text you are reading very quickly to get an overview of what the text is about, you do not need to read every word. You are probably doing it with this book without even realizing it.

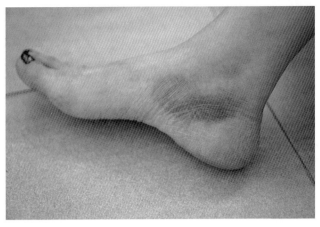

Fig. 3.1 Ouchy ankle.

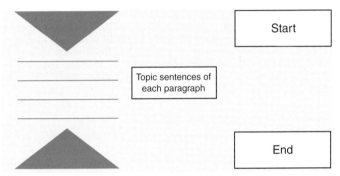

Fig. 3.2 Topic sentences.

To help with this you can:

- Look at headings, subheadings and summaries; for example, in this book you could look at the chapter titles or the information boxes at the top of the page
- Read the topic sentence of each paragraph (Fig. 3.2; this is usually the first sentence, which gives you an overview of what the paragraph is about). If it's not useful, move on

Some examples of topic sentences are:

- Drugs can be administered through a range of different routes. This includes orally, intravenously, inhalation and sublingual. For each of these routes there are a range of different factors that can influence the rate of absorption.
- Freddie and Madison were the first paramedics on the scene at the gas explosion. There were 20 to 30 workers who were thought to be trapped in the clothing factory.

The first sentence usually gives you an idea of what the paragraph will be about. You can see if it is what you are looking for and, if not, move on. You can tell that these two examples are from different texts.

Scanning the text means looking for a particular piece of information you have in mind. If you are looking at a printed book, you can use the index and table of contents. If you are scanning an e-book or the PDF of a journal article, you can use the search tool and type in the key word to help find the relevant section.

For example, if you want to find out about the blood and its components you could check the index for 'blood' or 'circulatory system' or type these terms into the search bar.

If you have dyslexia you might find it helpful to use a coloured overlay or a reading ruler to help you with your reading. You can also change the colour of the screen on your computer if you are reading online; there are lots of free screen tinting downloads once you know which colours work for you.

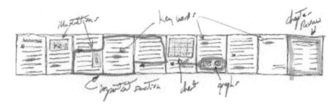

Fig. 3.3 Reading scroll.

READING SCROLLS

This is a technique developed by David Middlebrook (Middlebrook 1994). You can make a journal article or book chapter into a reading scroll. This enables you to get an overview of the entire thing and see it as a whole.

For example, you will be able to see the abstract and all the headings at once, which you couldn't by only looking at one page at a time. It also gives you the chance to mark them, highlighting the key information.

1. Start by printing out a journal article (one-sided) and sellotaping all of the pages together to make a scroll.
2. Next, skim through the text, identifying relevant features, and mark them on the text. This could be the abstract, results table or summary of the findings. You could also make notes on the side relating the text to your assignment.
3. Then draw a box around the features you have identified. This will make the most useful information stand out. Highlighter pens will help with this. We like to use different colours for different sections of my work; using the example of the ankle fracture, for instance, we would use blue for the introduction information (like general information about fractures), then pink to cover the current treatment, then green for possible alternatives and finally yellow for evidence.

You can see that, on this scroll, it is easy to pick out the most useful parts of the text (Fig. 3.3).

To find out more about reading scrolls you can visit the Textmapping project website: http://www.textmapping.org/unrollingTheBook.html.

APPROACHING A MORE DIFFICULT TEXT

Some of the texts that you need to read may seem very complicated. There are two strategies that you can use to help you with this:

- One is **prereading**—this means that before you approach a more difficult text you do some background research on the topic; in other words, find about the topic so you go into it with a bit more understanding. You could do this in a number of ways, such as watching a YouTube video (there are some really good videos out there) or having a look back through your lecture notes.
- Another similar strategy is **dual reading**, where you refer to an easier-to-read text just before reading a more difficult one. I really like this technique, but try them all and see what works for you.

Another technique is to have an introductory textbook on hand to look up anything you don't understand in a difficult journal article.

> Consider using books outside the reading list because they are often more understandable. Lecturers have a habit of putting the more complex books on the list, rather than the easy-to-understand ones. There is nothing wrong with starting with a basic human anatomy book, just make sure you progress to the reading list books.

Alternatively, you can use programs such as Read and Write or the Immersive Reader tool in Microsoft Office to read the article to you. You can pause it when you don't understand something or play it over until it starts to make sense. A lot of university libraries have facilities to do this; if you need some help, you just have to ask.

The Immersive Reader tool in Microsoft Office (Word) is easy to use and it is on most computers now. Just go into the Review menu, highlight the text and click on 'Read aloud speech—as circled', and the computer will read it to you. The voice is a little tinny-sounding, but it will do the job. Obviously (or not) you can copy and paste the article into Word if you do not have another option available to you and the article is in another format (Fig. 3.4).

> Prioritize your reading by only reading what you have to to answer the question—scan it to make sure it's relevant before reading the whole thing, otherwise you will just get word-blind, and nothing will make sense.
> Don't waste your time!

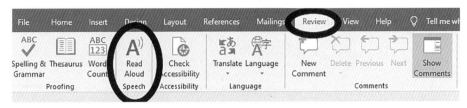

Fig. 3.4 The Immersive Reader: Word.

NOTE TAKING

First of all, you must decide if you need to take notes. Consider their purpose: if you are just making your classroom notes neat to put in a folder and never use again, then rewriting them is a waste of time. However, if you need to use them to revise or to use information in your assignments, go ahead. Studying is time consuming, so don't do things you don't have to.

Some universities are now recording the lecture and then publishing the link for you to use. Consider if this will work for you instead. Alternatively, annotating PowerPoint demonstrations can often be just as good as note taking because it will remind you of the lecture.

If you do need to take notes, then there are lots of different ways of doing this. You can try lots of different strategies until you find a strategy that works best for you.

It is important that your notes are usable and that you do actually go back and refer to them. To do this, you need to have a system for making notes. This could be storing them in a paper file or organizing them electronically into the relevant folder on your computer or tablet.

It is also helpful if your notes are relatively short and if you write in your own words, rather than copying out large sections of other people's text. Don't just copy from the text or from the lectures slides because lecturers often give you a lot more information than what is on the screen. If you want large pieces of information, you might as well make a note of the book or journal rather than copying it all out.

> Do not just copy out what it says in the book. When you come back to your notes you need to be able to tell what are your ideas and words and what are the authors' because you might accidentally commit plagiarism.
>
> Make sure you note down the full referencing details of any information you store so it will be easier to compile your reference list at the end of your work.

MIND MAPPING

1. Start by writing the central idea in a bubble in the middle of the page
2. Add related ideas as branches
3. Make connection between the ideas by drawing lines between them
4. You can add images or symbols to highlight key aspects of the map

You can now get mind-mapping software, which makes it easier to create a mind map and move the ideas around. Sometimes your university will have this available for students to use. Inspiration is one program I have used successfully in the past.

KEYWORD NOTES

You can do this by hand by getting a set of index cards, or you can open a PowerPoint file. Just write the keyword down, and then add all the relevant notes associated with it.

For example:

The skeletal system—206 bones (not including the bones of the ear)—split into appendicular skeleton and axial skeleton function—support, protection, movement, blood production...

CORNELL NOTES

This note-taking system (Cornell University) is particularly useful to use when you are revising for an exam. Start by dividing the piece of paper into three columns (Fig. 3.5):

- **Cue column**—needs to include keywords and any questions; completed after lectures
- **Note column**—includes main lecture notes, abbreviations, key thoughts and diagrams (leave a space between topics); written during lectures
  Summary—highlights the key points; written after lectures

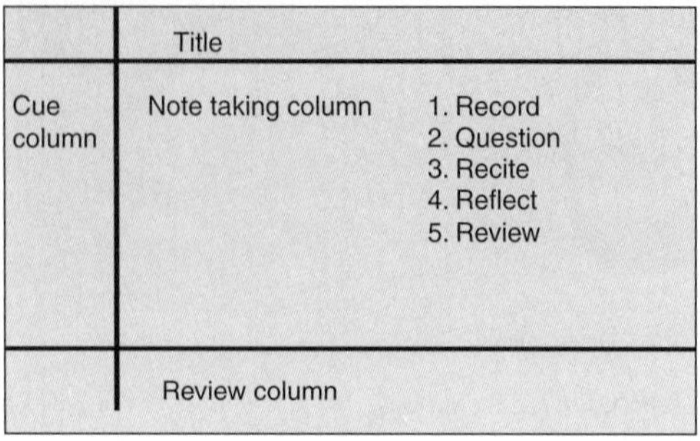

	Title	
Cue column	Note taking column	1. Record 2. Question 3. Recite 4. Reflect 5. Review
	Review column	

Fig. 3.5 Cornell notes.

REFERENCES

Cornell University. (U.D). The Cornell note taking system [Online]. Available at: http://lsc.cornell.edu/study-skills/cornell-note-taking-system/. Accessed on 01/08/2020.

Middlebrook, R. D. (1994). Using scrolls [Online]. Available at: http://www.textmapping.org/using.html. Accessed on 31/07/2020.

REFERENCING

CHAPTER 4

CHAPTER OUTLINE

SO WHEN DO YOU NEED TO INCLUDE A REFERENCE?
WHAT IS GOOD EVIDENCE?
Journal Articles
Websites
REFERENCING YOUR WORK
In-Text Citations
Sources in the Reference List
Referencing a Book
Referencing a Journal Article
Referencing a Report

A Reference List or Bibliography
REFERENCE MANAGEMENT SOFTWARE
WAYS OF USING EVIDENCE
Direct Quote
SUMMARY
Paraphrase
INTRODUCING A SOURCE
CHAPTER SUMMARY

OVERVIEW:

- This chapter starts by looking at when you need to include references in your work.
- Next, we will consider what we mean by 'good evidence', as well as the different types of sources you might refer to during your degree.
- Following on from this we will look at the principles of referencing and how to reference using the Harvard style.
- Finally, we will review the different ways of including evidence in your assignment: referencing, paraphrasing and summarizing.

As we have seen in Chapter 2, supporting our points with evidence is one of the features that makes our work academic, and it is important if you want to pass.

An example of this might be that you are writing an essay about the use of collars in penetrating lower back trauma, and you think that they can cause more problems to the patient, including putting pressure on the vagus nerve, which will slow the patient's respiratory rate. It is all well and good saying it, but your lecturers will need evidence to support your view, and trust us, there is evidence out there: you just have to find it and reference it, making sure it's from a good source (not *Paramedics Weekly* by Fred the want-to-be part-time paramedic…ok, that's made up, but you get what we mean).

This means that your whole process of writing will be different to what you have used before attending university because you need to factor in researching and referencing. However, once you get used to this, it will be a lot easier and almost second nature: so bear with it!

Although the advice in this chapter will be useful to all student paramedics and allied healthcare professionals, each university will have a preferred system of referencing, so you should check with your lecturers which one they want you to use.

Most universities use plagiarism software packages such as Turnitin. These will check the similarity of your work to books or published articles, as well as other students' work. Each program will then generate a similarity score and show the lecturer the exact sources your text came from. It is a robust system, so you must reference unless you want to end up in front of an academic offences panel.

You can also ask one of your university librarians (Fig. 4.1) for help with referencing and finding information because they will know what sources are available to you, and often which are the best to use. They really are a good source of knowledge for everything academic, so make sure you use them and do not overlook them.

SO WHEN DO YOU NEED TO INCLUDE A REFERENCE?

You need to include a reference whenever you refer to something you have read. This will show that you aren't trying to tell the lecturer that the work is just yours; it also adds validity to what you are writing.

This does not just apply when you have used a direct quote: you also need to reference things you have summarized (read a paragraph and written a shorter version of it) and paraphrased (used the same information, just changing a couple of words here and there).

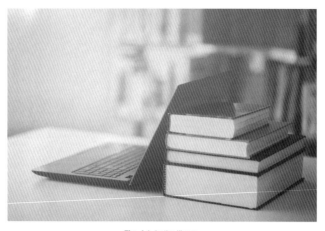

Fig. 4.1 In the library.

Because all healthcare degrees are evidence-based, you will need to provide a reference every time you claim something is a fact. This may mean that you need to look for a reference for something that you already know. A good rule of thumb is that if you are in doubt it is best to provide a reference.

WHAT IS GOOD EVIDENCE?

It is important that you are selective about the types of evidence that you use and only use things from reliable sources. You should avoid using websites such as Wikipedia where it is not clear who the author is. Most of the information you will refer to in your degree should come from academic sources, as listed later. The best way to find this type of material is by searching on your university library website or through Google Scholar, the part of Google that only searches for academic research. Just doing an ordinary Google (or any other search engine) search is not going to get you the right sort of material for university-level work. Some of the main types of sources you will use are (Fig. 4.2):

- Journal articles
- Books
- Websites
- Government reports
- Research reports

Here, we will look at each source of evidence.

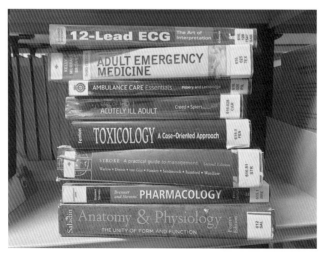

Fig. 4.2 Journals, books, computers; it goes on and on.

Journal Articles

A journal article is usually a report of a single piece of research. Journal articles are considered to be a reliable source of information because to be published, they have to go through a process known as peer review. This means that experts in that subject have reviewed the article without knowing who the authors are to decide if it is of a high enough standard to be published and if any changes need to be made.

Journal articles tend to be very specific. They are also written for an audience of researchers, so can be quite difficult to understand (Fig. 4.3). It might be a good idea to start looking at journals only after you have got a good overview of the topic from other sources.

The structure of journal articles is as follows:

- **Title**—the article will have a title telling you exactly what the research is about. Sometimes students confuse this with the title of the journal. Make sure you know the difference; the title will be the first large piece of writing you will come to. The title of the journal will be written in a smaller font at the top or bottom of the page.
- **Abstract**—most journal articles start with an abstract. This is a one-paragraph summary of the research. It should contain information about the background to the research, the methods they used and what they found. You should get a sense if the article is going to be useful to you just from the abstract, so you don't have to waste your time reading the whole article if it's not relevant.
- **Everything else**—the rest of the article includes the methodology, which is how they undertook the study and research; the findings, which is what they actually discovered when they undertook the study; and then a discussion, which draws conclusions from the study. Often the discussion will include limitations of the study; for example, a small number of participants (a small sample size) or anything else that might need to be taken into consideration when looking at the study results.

Websites

There is a lot of useful information on the internet. However, as you must be aware, there is also a load of rubbish, including some health advice that is actually dangerous and just not true.

Because no one would want the clinician who is responsible for saving their life to have got his or her information from somewhere dodgy on the internet (remember *Paramedic Weekly* by Fred? well, websites can be similar), it is important to think critically about the sources that you use. Ask yourself: can I trust this source? Who has written it?

For example, the British Heart Foundation's information on heart attacks is going to be trustworthy (but may be aimed at the general public rather than health professionals). Have a look at these types of websites; there is often a tab for healthcare professionals—yep, that's you now.

As a general rule, if you can find the information in a more academic source (books or journal articles), then use those instead. Websites may have the most up-to-date information for certain topics, and they do have their place, so don't disregard them.

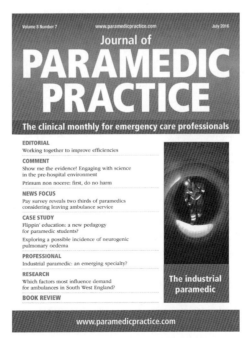

Fig. 4.3 *Journal of Paramedic Practice.*

Wikipedia is not considered a good academic source because it is not generally peer-reviewed—stay away. Also, make sure you don't reference search engines such as Bing or Google—we've seen it happen.

REFERENCING YOUR WORK

So now that we have looked at the types of references you can use, you need to understand how to put them into your work.

Most university paramedic and allied healthcare courses will specify that you use Harvard referencing or a close variation to this, so this is what we will use in the examples later. There are some common elements that you need to include in all referencing systems which will allow the reader to understand where you got the sources of information to write your assignment.

You need to remember that at universities it is not just essays that need referencing: it is any piece of academic work you do where you have used information sources. This might include posters, presentations and essays, just to name a few.

There are two main components to Harvard referencing that you need to get to grips with:

- **A citation in the text.** This is used within your work where you have put information in from another source, which can be anything from a television show to a book, a journal or even a person. This just gives the author's last name and the date, for example, '(Jones, 2018)'. If it is from an alternative source, for example, the government website, the main source is listed instead of the author name, for example, '(GOV.UK, 2019)'.
- **A reference list at the end of your work.** This gives the full source information. Be aware that all academic work will require a reference list, and everything that you have referenced in the text must appear in the reference list.

The idea is that you should be able to match the citation in the text to the full reference at the end, so that if someone wants to find the original source it is easy for them to do so.

It also ensures you give credit for the information to the right person and you don't try to pass the work off as your own.

Some universities have their own style of Harvard referencing, so make sure you check. Your library will be able to tell you the correct style to use and give you further guidance.

> Just a gentle reminder that there are many different types of referencing; you will need to check with your university which one they use.
> We have chosen to demonstrate the Harvard style of referencing because it is one of the most frequently used throughout universities; however, most styles follow a similar pattern.

In-Text Citations

There are two ways of doing an in-text citation. If the author's name is part of the text, only the date is in the brackets; for example, 'according to Khan (2019)…'.

If their name is not part of the sentence, then you write your summary or paraphrase and then put the name and date just after: 'Hip fractures are more common in people with osteoporosis' (NHS, 2020).

If you are citing a source that has more than three authors, you just give the name of the first author and then 'et al.' (this is Latin for 'and others'). In the full referencing list at the end you give the names of all the authors (but this can vary, so check your guide). For example: '(Davis et al., 2017)'.

Some of the sources you use won't have a named author, so instead you will cite the organization that produced it, for example, National Health Service (NHS), College of Paramedics, National Institute for Health and Care Excellence, and so on. If there is no date (as is often the case for websites), just write 'no date' in parentheses.

Sources in the Reference List

The key to writing a good reference list is to think about what type of source it is and follow the format for that type of source. This sounds easy, but many people reference a journal article as they would a website, because they accessed it on the internet, but this is not right.

Referencing a Book

When you reference a book, you need to think about how many authors there are and if it is an edited book where different chapters are written by different authors.

If the book just has one author you would reference it like this:
Author Surname, Initial(s). (Year). *Title*. Edition (if not first edition). Place of publication: Publisher.
For example:
Collen, A. (2017). *Decision Making in Paramedic Practice*. Bridgwater: Class Publishing.
However, if there are two or three authors it would be like this:
Author Surname, Initial(s). and Author Surname, Initial(s). (Year). *Title*. Edition (if not first edition). Place of publication: Publisher.
For example:
Blaber, A. and Harris, G. (2016). *Assessment Skills for Paramedics*. 2nd ed. Maidenhead: Open University Press.
If there are more than three authors, you would usually just write the name of the first author and then 'et al.'. However, this is different in different versions of Harvard, so check with your university.

REFERENCING **23**

If you are referencing a chapter of an edited book, then you need to give the name of the author who wrote the chapter first, then the title of the chapter and the full details of the book following the format below:

Chapter Author Surname, Initial(s). (Year). Title of chapter. In Editor(s) Initial(s). Editor(s) Surname, ed(s)., *Title of Book*, Edition (if not first). Place of publication: Publisher, Page numbers.

For example:

Cox, N. (2016). Cardiovascular system. In T. A., Roper, ed., *Clinical Skills,* 2nd ed. Oxford: Oxford University Press, pp 28-83.

REFERENCING A JOURNAL ARTICLE

Most journal articles should be referenced following this format. Note that it is the title of the journal, not the article itself, that is in italics.

Author Surname, Initial(s). (Year). Title of article. *Full Title of Journal*, Volume number(Issue/Part number), Page number(s).

For example:

Ennis, P. (2019). A pilot of the Paramedic Advanced Resuscitation of Children (PARC) course. *Journal of Paramedic Practice*, 11(11), 470–478.

Some journals that are available in an online format have something called a digital object identifier (DOI). If this is the case, you will need to give the DOI number as well (unsurprisingly, it is a number that starts with 'DOI').

Author Surname, Initial(s). (Year). Title of article. *Full Title of Journal,* [online] Volume(Issue), pages. Available at: URL including DOI [Accessed Day Mo. Year].

For example:

Izawa J, Komukai S, Gibo K, Okubo M, Kiyohara K, Nishiyama C et al. Pre-hospital advanced airway management for adults with out-of-hospital cardiac arrest: nationwide cohort study BMJ 2019;364:l430. https://doi.org/10.1136/bmj.l430

REFERENCING A REPORT

Often reports have what is sometimes referred to as a 'corporate author'. This means that it has been written by an organization such as the NHS or the Department of Health rather than a named individual.

Physical item

Author Surname, Initial(s). or Corporate Author. (Year of publication). *Title of report.* Report number [if applicable]. Place of Publication: Publisher.

College of Paramedics. (2018). *Practice Guidance for Paramedics for the Administration of Medicines Under Exemptions Within the Human Medicines Regulations 2012.* V0.13. Bridgwater: College of Paramedics.

Online/electronic

Author Surname, Initial(s). or Corporate Author. (Year of publication). *Title of report.* Paper number [if applicable] [online]. Place of Publication: Publisher. Available at: URL or DOI. [Date Viewed].

Department of Health. (2015). *Mental Health Act 1983: Code of Practice* [online]. London: The Stationery Office. Available at: https://assets.publishing.service.gov.uk/government/uploads/system/uploads/attachment_data/file/435512/MHA_Code_of_Practice.PDF. [Accessed 17 Apr. 2020].

A REFERENCE LIST OR BIBLIOGRAPHY

A reference list is a list of everything that you have cited in the assignment. Sometimes you may be asked to provide a bibliography, which is a list of everything you have read. It is in the same format as a reference list, but you also include what you have read but not actually cited in the assignment. For both reference lists and bibliographies, you will need to list all the sources in alphabetical order based on the author's last name.

Example reference list:

References:

Blaber, A and Harris, G. (2016). *Assessment skills for paramedics* 2nd ed. Maidenhead: Open University Press.

College of Paramedics. (2018). *Practice Guidance for Paramedics for the Administration of Medicines Under Exemptions Within the Human Medicines Regulations 2012.* V0.13. Bridgwater: College of Paramedics.

Collen, A. (2017). *Decision Making in Paramedic Practice.* Bridgwater: Class Publishing.

Cox, N. (2016). Cardiovascular system. In: T. A. Roper, ed., *Clinical Skills,* 2nd ed. Oxford: Oxford University Press, pp 28-83.

Department of Health. (2015). *Mental Health Act 1983: Code of Practice* [online]. London: The Stationery Office. Available at: https://assets.publishing.service.gov.uk/government/uploads/system/uploads/attachment_data/file/435512/MHA_Code_of_Practice.PDF. [Accessed 17 Apr. 2020].

Ennis, P. (2019). A pilot of the Paramedic Advanced Resuscitation of Children (PARC) course. *Journal of Paramedic Practice*, 11(11).

Izawa, J., et al. (2019). Pre-hospital advanced airway management for adults with out-of-hospital cardiac arrest: nationwide cohort study. *British Medical Journal,* 364():l430. Available at: https://doi.org/10.1136/bmj.l430. [Accessed 17 Apr. 2020].

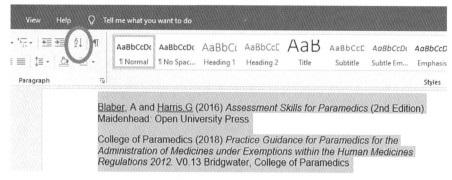

Blaber, A and Harris,G (2016) *Assessment Skills for Paramedics* (2nd Edition) Maidenhead: Open University Press

College of Paramedics (2018) *Practice Guidance for Paramedics for the Administration of Medicines under Exemptions within the Human Medicines Regulations 2012*. V0.13 Bridgwater, College of Paramedics

Fig. 4.4 Alphabetical ordering.

> To put your reference list in order, you can use the sort A–Z function in Microsoft Word (found on the Home tab). Highlight the entire list and press the button. Alternatively, you can use the reference management software (as described later) to help you organize your reference list (Fig. 4.4).

REFERENCE MANAGEMENT SOFTWARE

You may find it helpful to use a reference management software program to keep track of your references. These programs can store all your references in one place and make it easier for you to add them into your text and create a bibliography at the end. There are some reference management software programs that can be downloaded for free by anyone, such as Mendeley and Zotero.

Your university may also subscribe to a paid service. This can be really useful because there will be some support available for using it. Have a look on your university's library website or ask someone to find out. Refworks is one that is often used within libraries and can automatically save references from Google Scholar searches.

Microsoft Word also has a referencing package that is fairly easy to use. You will need to type in the information from the reference, but it will formulate the reference list and you only have to enter the reference once (Fig. 4.5).

WAYS OF USING EVIDENCE

There are three main ways of including evidence in your writing: as a summary, a paraphrase or a direct quote. Whichever type you use, you still need to put a reference in the text as outlined above. Some students think that they don't need to put a reference in if they rewrite something in their own words, but this is wrong: you do need to put a reference.

DIRECT QUOTE

Direct quotes should be used sparingly, but they are useful for definitions. You need to use the exact words that the author did, and also give the page number.

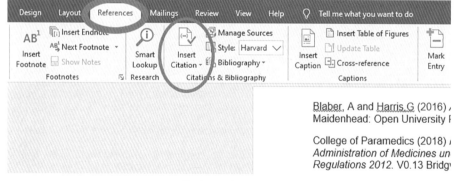

Fig. 4.5 Inserting citations.

For example:

> *"Everyone who works in healthcare works extremely hard, but the rewards are also vast; although the vast majority of workers think they should have a large pay rise so they can retire early and travel the world on a big red and green boat"* (Cobb et al., 2020, p. 72).

SUMMARY

Most of the time when you reference you will be using a summary or a direct quote. When you do this, you will use your own words. Most universities now ask students to submit their work through a text-matching software called Turnitin. This means that the wording will have to be significantly different from the original source. This is easier when writing a summary because what you are saying is much shorter than the original source. The idea is to give the main points of a much larger text (or even more than one text) in one or two sentences.

To write an effective summary, read the original until you are familiar with it. It is often easier to write the summary from memory rather than looking at the original text. Only include the main points that are relevant to your assignment—you don't need to summarize the whole source if it is not relevant.

PARAPHRASE

Paraphrasing is when you rewrite an idea in your own words.

Example text:

The follow-up questionnaire revealed that the majority of the seven paramedics responding had been required to deal with an emergency involving a child since the course, with only one reporting that they had not. All those who had attended a children's emergency reported they felt more confident in dealing with the incident as a result of having attended the course.

A bad example of paraphrasing:

Six out of the seven paramedics who responded to the survey had been required to deal with an emergency involving a child since the training. Everyone who had attended a children's emergency said they felt more confident in dealing with it as a result of the course (Ennis, 2019).

This has exactly the same order and phrases as the original source.

A good example of paraphrase:

Ennis (2019) followed up the training session with a survey. All six of the paramedics responding who had dealt with a call involving a child reported that attending the course had given them more confidence in handling the situation.

This is much better. It is written in the student's own style.

Top tips for paraphrasing:

- Change the order that you present the information in
- Where you can, change the words or use different forms of words
- Use different sentence structures

INTRODUCING A SOURCE

The language you use to introduce a piece of evidence can let us know what you think of it. For example, 'Jones (2018) established that…' suggests that you agree with what they say and are confident that it is right. If you were to write 'Smith (2012) suggests that…', this would imply you were more cautious about what they were saying.

Some good reporting verbs to use are:

- Comments
- Claims
- Argues
- States
- Demonstrates

CHAPTER SUMMARY

- It is vital to use up-to-date evidence in your writing
- This means you need to do a lot of reading; but be selective about what you read
- Every time you claim something is a fact you need to include a reference
- There are different styles of referencing, and you need to make sure you use the one that is accepted on your course
- You can include evidence as a summary, paraphrase or direct quote

REFERENCES

Blaber, A. & Harris, G. (2016). *Assessment skills for paramedics*, 2nd ed. Maidenhead: Open University Press.

College of Paramedics. (2018). *Practice guidance for paramedics for the administration of medicines under exemptions within the human medicines regulations 2012*. V0.13 Bridgwater: College of Paramedics.

Collen, A. (2017). *Decision making in paramedic practice*. Bridgwater: Class Publishing.

Cox, N. (2016). Cardiovascular system. In: T. A. Roper, ed., *Clinical skills*, (2nd ed). Oxford: Oxford University Press, pp 28-83.

Department of Health. (2015). *Mental Health Act 1983: Code of Practice* [Online]. London: The Stationery Office. Available at: https://assets. publishing.service.gov.uk/government/uploads/system/uploads/attachment_data/file/435512/MHA_Code_of_Practice.PDF. Accessed on 17/04/2020.

Ennis, P. (2019). A pilot of the Paramedic Advanced Resuscitation of Children (PARC) course. *Journal of Paramedic Practice*, 11(11).

Izawa, J., et al. (2019). Pre-hospital advanced airway management for adults with out-of-hospital cardiac arrest: nationwide cohort study. *British Medical Journal,* 364, l430. Available at: https://doi.org/10.1136/bmj.l430. Accessed on 17/04/2020.

CHAPTER 5

RESEARCH METHODS AND LITERATURE SEARCHING

CHAPTER OUTLINE

IN THIS CHAPTER:

- We introduce you to the types of research that you might come across in your studies.
- We tell you how to do a basic literature search.
- We look at how to do a systematic literature search, including developing a structured question.
- Finally, we discuss how to critically appraise sources, including using different frameworks.

RESEARCH: THE BASICS

As a paramedic and a healthcare professional, it is vital to make sure that the care you give is underpinned by the best possible evidence. To do this, you need to understand the research evidence and know how to find it, so that if you ever end up in front of the HCPC or in the coroner's court you can justify your actions with research. We are not going to go into a lot of depth about the different research methods (there are lots of good books on those), but will get you to a point where you can read a journal article and make sense of it.

You will hear the term 'evidence-based practice' both in university and, increasingly, when you are out and about actually doing your job. This term means exactly what it says: you base your practice on actual evidence.

An example of this might be something like when to put in an I-gel or an ET tube. You have looked at the research that has been undertaken, and you have identified that neither advanced airway was discovered to be favourable when it came to patient outcome. However, the findings identified there were more potential complications with ET tubes (Benger et al. 2018), and therefore you decide to use an I-gel rather than an ET tube where clinically possible. This is **evidence-based practice.**

Bear in mind what we said in Chapter 4 (if you have not looked, it is all about referencing) that no matter how much you know about a topic you still might find things you need to look up. This is when you read a journal article or another form of literature.

Researching is a systematic approach to gathering information, with the aim of gaining new knowledge. A systematic approach is something that is organized: you follow the steps, which will lead you to the best possible information.

There are many different types of studies. Some of these are listed here, but the main areas that these fall into are primary and secondary research. Primary research is research that has been undertaken directly, such as the AIRWAYS trial we discuss later because the study was undertaken by paramedics on the ground.

Secondary research is also valid research, but it gathers existing data rather than generating new data. So it might gather data regarding something like prevalence of secondary strokes and then analyse them in relation to a particular treatment that is already being used, such as a nurse-led intervention service. The recurrence rates could then be compared with those observed in a trust that does not currently have the same type of service. The data are then collated and analysed, and conclusions about the effectiveness of the intervention service are drawn.

WHAT IS THE LITERATURE?

You will often hear your lectures referring to the literature. This just means the previous research that has been done on your topic. There are lots of different types of literature, and they can all be used, as long as you can demonstrate the validity of the research (that it is factually sound). This is a skill we will talk about later.

QUALITATIVE AND QUANTITATIVE RESEARCH

There are two main types of research: qualitative and quantitative (within these there is a huge variety of different types of methods). Some studies use a mixture of qualitative and quantitative research methods, and this approach is referred to, strangely enough, as mixed methods.

These two approaches represent different paradigms; a paradigm is a shared understanding that scientists have about what we know about the world and everything in it. The two different paradigms are just to different ways we get this understanding.

When evaluating research, you need to consider if the approach taken was appropriate for the question being investigated because each different paradigm is best suited to different types of research questions.

QUALITATIVE RESEARCH

The term 'qualitative research' refers to any type of research that collects nonnumerical data. Qualitative research tends to focus on the human and interpersonal side of healthcare; because of this, it can be easier to relate to and understand. Qualitative methods are suited to research that aims to find out about people's lived experiences in their own words. Unlike quantitative research, qualitative research can allow for some subjectivity.

An example of qualitative research is a paper entitled 'Women's experience of unplanned out of hospital birth in paramedic care' (Flanagan et al. 2019) which reported that, while paramedics often care for women in labour, it is much less common for them to be there for the birth. However, research has identified that in Australia 92% of out-of-hospital births were attended by paramedics.

Although there was existing research on the clinical factors that might lead to women having an unplanned birth out of the hospital, as well as the outcomes for mother and baby, there was not very much known about the women's personal experiences. This is important because it has been previously identified in research that a woman's birth experience has an impact on her overall wellbeing.

The researchers carried out narrative interviews with 22 women in Queensland, Australia who had given birth outside of the hospital in the care of paramedics. The women were prompted to give an account of their birth experience. A thematic analysis of all the participants' accounts was carried out.

The research found that whether women had a positive or negative birth experience was largely attributed to their perception of the paramedics' communication skills, highlighting the importance of patient-centred care. It highlighted some concerns about consent not being obtained for certain procedures. This type of information would be difficult to obtain from quantitative research.

QUANTITATIVE RESEARCH

Quantitative research is the type of research that we associate most with the traditional scientific methods. It adopts a positivist paradigm (objective reality against which researchers can compare their claims and ascertain truth), where data is collected in a format that can be measured and statistically analysed.

An example of quantitative research is the paper entitled 'Effect of a Strategy of a Supraglottic Airway Device vs Tracheal Intubation During Out-of-Hospital Cardiac Arrest on Functional Outcome: The AIRWAYS-2 Randomized Clinical Trial' (Benger et al. 2018). This study investigated whether using a supraglottic airway device (SGA) for advanced airway management was more effective than using tracheal intubation (TI) for patients who had a nontraumatic out-of-hospital cardiac arrest.

This was a randomized clinical trial involving paramedics from four different ambulance services. It was considered to be too complex to randomize the participants, so the paramedics were randomly allocated airway management strategies, with 764 paramedics allocated TI and 759 SGA. The allocation was done using computer software. All patients over 18 years who had an out-of-hospital cardiac arrest (9296 in total) were enrolled in the study by a consent waiver, as it would not be possible to obtain their consent at the time.

The researchers used the modified Rankin score as a measure of how effective the treatment was. A Rankin score of 0 to 3 signifies a good outcome, and a score of 4 to 6 signifies a poor outcome/death. The data were subjected to a range of statistical tests, including mixed effects logistic regression. This difference was not high enough to be statistically significant. As this research was investigating the effectiveness of the treatment, a quantitative approach involving a large number of patients was needed. It was important to use a measure of success that could be measured numerically so that statistical analysis could be done to determine which approach was more effective.

You can see that the methods used for each of the research examples, although very different, were appropriate for the research question. For most medical research, a quantitative approach would be the most relevant. A large sample size is better because you are more likely to be able to generalize.

If you are not sure if the piece of research that you are reading is qualitative or quantitative, have a look at the results. If the authors have presented a lot of statistics, then it is most likely quantitative; if they have presented a lot of quotes from

Table 5.1 Differences Between Qualitative and Quantitative Research

QUALITATIVE RESEARCH	QUANTITATIVE RESEARCH
Concerned about finding about people's lived experiences, from their own perspective	Aims to find out facts about the world
Interpretivist paradigm	Positivist paradigm
Does not use statistical analysis	Uses statistical analysis
Sample population is normally small	Sample population is often large
Data collection methods are semistructured	Data collection methods are highly structured

research participants, then it is qualitative. If a study has a mixture of both of these, then it was probably a mixed methods study (the third research type).

Table 5.1 summarizes the differences between the two types of research.

DIFFERENT TYPES OF JOURNAL ARTICLES

When looking at research it is important to know about the different types of journal articles you might come across. Whereas most journal articles report a single piece of original research, not all of them do. There are some other types of articles as described here.

- **Case studies:** These look at lived experience or examples of real-life events.
- **Reviews:** These can be narrative or systematic reviews, as well as metaanalyses, which examine lots of data on the same subject from independent sources to determine any patterns (or trends).
- **Opinion piece/perspective piece:** Some journals have a section which allows practitioners or researchers to present their opinions. As with all research, you will need to consider the validity of these pieces (this means asking whether the practitioner or researcher is experienced or qualified enough to give informed information). Consider us as paramedics writing an article on quantum physics: this would not be considered valid, because, believe it or not, we know nothing about quantum physics.

THE HIERARCHY OF EVIDENCE

When you are looking at evidence to include in your work, you need to consider the hierarchy of evidence. This can be considered the scale of the best possible evidence down to *Uncle Bob's Home-Written Journal of Trains*. Fig. 5.1 shows a pyramid of evidence, with the top being considered the best (most valid).

Glover et al. (2006) Evidence-Based Medicine Pyramid

There are some different variants of the hierarchy. The Oxford Centre for Evidence-Based Medicine (2011) uses a table with questions to structure their hierarchy of evidence. For most of the questions, systematic reviews are still the most effective forms of evidence. However, the authors are more critical about relying on the judgement of other clinicians, as they argue that too much weight can be put on the opinions of the researchers, and that clinicians should exercise their own clinical judgement. Healthcare professionals still need to consider if a study has been carried out well.

Here are the different types of research contained in the hierarchy:

- **Opinion piece:** Some journals have a section which allows practitioners or researchers to present their opinions. This is often in an area where there is not an established base of research, and may suggest areas which researchers may want to pursue. This can give us insight into an expert's clinical experience; but, of course, this is just one person's view.
- **Case study:** A case study is a description of an individual case, the intervention and the outcome. This may be useful for a scenario that is very rare but because it is only based on one person, few generalizations can be made. A case series will include a series of case studies. For example, Zhang et al. (2020) identified all four known cases of the novel coronavirus in babies under 28 days old and described their symptoms, treatment and prognosis. This was useful because there was very little known about how the virus affects babies.
- **Cohort study:** Cohort studies follow two groups of patients over a period of time and compare them. For example, this could be one group of patients with a risk factor for a particular medical condition and a control group of individuals who don't have this risk factor. This gives us the chance to see how the cases progress.
- **Randomized control trial:** This is a type of study which randomly allocates participants to one of two groups to reduce the risk of bias. One group will receive the treatment, and one group will serve as a control (receiving either a well-established treatment or no treatment). Double-blind randomized control trials, where neither the patients nor the researchers know which group the patients have been allocated to, are considered to be more reliable because this study design eliminates any placebo effect on the side of the patient or bias on the side of the researchers. However, this is obviously only possible for certain types of treatment.

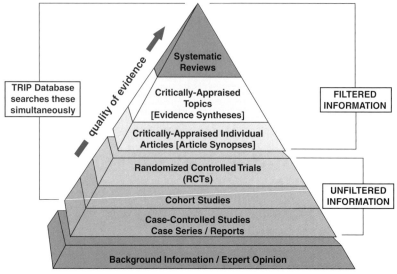

Fig. 5.1 Evidence-based pyramid.

- **Systematic review:** Systematic reviews aim to identify all previous research that has been done on a topic and produce a summary of the current state of knowledge. These differ from a standard literature review in that the authors go through a very structured process to ensure all the relevant literature is identified. This starts with a clearly defined research question. The researchers then search the literature and critically appraise the studies, making recommendations based on the best evidence. A **metaanalysis** is a type of systematic review which incorporates a statistical analysis of the results from all of the studies. Systematic reviews are considered to be a particularly rigorous form of research, as they are based on evidence from multiple research projects. However, sometimes the systematic review will not come up with a clear answer as to whether a treatment is effective. In this case you will need to refer back to the individual research articles included in the review to see what they found.

UNDERTAKING A BASIC LITERATURE SEARCH

Now that you understand the type of evidence you might find, you need to actually undertake your literature search.

If you want to do a literature search, there are two main sources that you might want to use. The first one will be your university library, because it will have a wide range of sources that you will have full access to.

If you want to supplement your library search, you can also try Google Scholar. This is an academic search engine that is part of Google (make sure it says scholar under the search bar; Fig. 5.2).

You will not have access to all the papers you find in Google Scholar, but it can take you to other sites where you may be able to get hold of some papers that your library doesn't have. Alternatively, if you find the paper in Google Scholar, get the information and speak to your library, they might be able to get hold of it for you, depending on the article and the university.

The first thing you need to do when you do a library search is to come up with some search terms. Think about what you want to find out, choose key words to describe your topic and consider whether there are any alternative words for your topic.

For example, if you are researching paramedics and end-of-life care you might want to use the key words PARAMEDICS and END OF LIFE CARE. This might identify 3000 articles or none at all, so you could add other words to your search to increase or decrease numbers. For example, you could put in PARAMEDICS or AMBULANCE and END OF LIFE CARE OR PALLIATIVE CARE.

LIMITATIONS

These are further ways of narrowing down the search to make sure you find something that you can actually use:
- **Time:** Databases and library search engines let you narrow down research to a particular time period. In most cases it is best to select research that has been carried out within the last 10 years. This means it is more up to date.

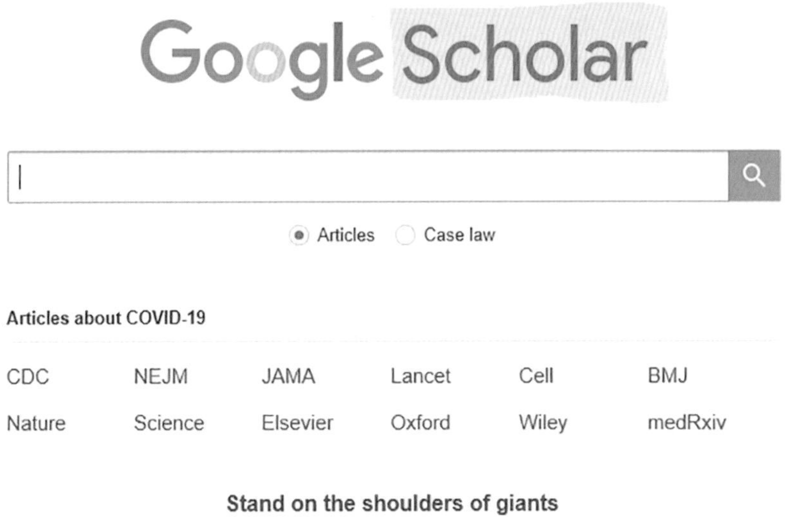

Google Scholar

	🔍

⦿ Articles ◯ Case law

Articles about COVID-19

CDC	NEJM	JAMA	Lancet	Cell	BMJ
Nature	Science	Elsevier	Oxford	Wiley	medRxiv

Stand on the shoulders of giants

Fig. 5.2 Google Scholar.

- **Language:** This allows you to choose the language you want the research to be in.
- **Location:** You can specify a location for the research; for example, do you only want to use research that has been carried out in the United Kingdom, or do you also want to find international articles? If you use international articles, consider the context. Sometimes the search engines do not do a good job in filtering out international articles, so have a look at the authors' affiliations to check where the researcher is based.
- **Peer review:** It is best to check the box for peer review because this means that the research has been checked for quality. You can also limit your search by the type of source; for example, only books or only journal articles.

To look at the limitations, you need to jump on to your university system and have a play with entering search terms and limiting the results. It's like anything: the more you practice, the better you get at it.

WHY DO A SYSTEMATIC REVIEW?

When you are given a piece of work to do you need to undertake a systematic review of the topic. This means that you undertake a literature search to find and look at all the different information you can find on the subject you are being asked to write about. This will enable you to put lots of information into your piece of work and be fully informed about what you are writing about. Think of it this way: if you were buying a new phone and you knew nothing about phones (okay, so imagine you haven't ever had one before: difficult, we know), instead of picking the first one you come to, it would be more sensible to look at lots of different phones and pick the one that best suits your needs. Well, it is the same when undertaking a literature search for a piece of work: if you use the first article you come to and don't look at other sources of information, you might not put the correct stuff in you essay—ummm yep, a big fat fail. (We have heard it said that 'fail' stands for First Attempt In Learning, but really, you are going to be paramedics and healthcare professionals: we don't tend to go with that fluffy stuff. A fail means redoing it and having less time to do other fun stuff like watch Ambulance or 24 Hours in A&E!)

DOING A SYSTEMATIC LITERATURE SEARCH

So, because we like diagrams, here is one to show you the whole process: Fig. 5.3.

STRUCTURED QUESTIONS

You are more likely to perform a successful search if you have a clear idea of what you are asking and what you want to find out. Structured questions are one way of making sure that you do this. Sometimes you will be asked to use one, especially if you are doing a systematic literature search. There are a few different frameworks you can use to help you write a structured question. Choose one that is a good fit for what you want to investigate.

One of these is the PICO framework, which stands for:
- Patient or Population or Problem
- Intervention or exposure
- Comparisons
- Outcome (optional depending on question)

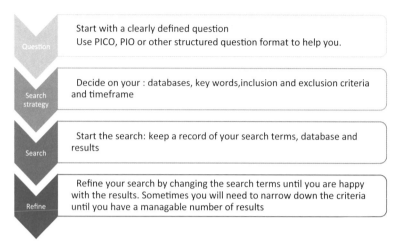

Fig. 5.3 Systemic literature search.

Imagine you wanted to research paramedic knowledge and training in providing suitable end-of-life care for dementia patients. You could use the following search terms:
- Population: dementia
- Intervention: end-of-life care
- Comparisons: skills and/or knowledge
- Outcome: as you are researching the outcome, you do not need to add this section

Or, if you are looking at whether the use of cannulation kits in ambulances rather than individual items that are stored loose can reduce infection rates at the site of cannulation, you could use the following search terms:
- Population: cannulated patients
- Intervention: use of sterile cannulation kits
- Comparison: individual items
- Outcome: reduced infection rates

SPIDER

This is the next searching framework you can use; it is mostly used when researching qualitative research.

This type of question allows you to focus on a particular healthcare setting, which makes it particularly useful for paramedics, where you want to find examples that relate to prehospital care.

SPIDER is an alternative to PICO that has a special focus on qualitative research (Cooke et al. 2012).

SPIDER framework
- **Sample:** The group of people being looked at. Because qualitative research is not easy to generalize, 'sample' is preferred over 'patient'.
- **Phenomenon of interest:** Looks at the reasons for behaviour and decisions, rather than an intervention.
- **Design:** The form of research used, such as interview or survey.
- **Evaluation:** The outcome measures.
- **Research type:** Qualitative, quantitative and/or mixed methods.

So let's look at the same examples we used earlier but apply the SPIDER framework to them.

You would like to research paramedic knowledge and training in providing suitable end-of-life care for dementia patients. You could use the following search terms:
- Sample: dementia patients
- Phenomenon of interest: skills and knowledge
- Design: interviews
- Evaluation: thematic analysis
- Research type: qualitative

A SEARCH STRATEGY

So, now that you have the knowledge of the searching framework, you need to undertake the search. First decide which database or databases you are going to use. Your university library will subscribe to a number of bibliographic healthcare databases. These are big collections of journal articles in different subject areas. Each one has a slightly different focus, so it is important to select the right one for your particular search or use a combination.

DATABASES

Some of the databases that are most useful for paramedics are:

> CINAHL (Cumulative Index to Nursing and Allied Health Literature)
> This is an international database which includes journal articles relating to nursing and allied health professionals.
>
> Science Direct
> This includes all of the journals published by Elsevier. The journals are grouped into four main sections: Physical Sciences and Engineering, Life Sciences, Health Sciences and Social Sciences and Humanities.
>
> Cochrane Library
> This is a database of evidence-based interventions in healthcare. It is free to access, so does not depend on your library having a subscription. The Cochrane Library is famous for its systematic literature reviews. It also has a section on randomized control trials and clinical answers.
>
> Medline and PubMed
> A medical database that searches the US National Library of Medicine. PubMed is the free version, whereas Medline is a subscription version that your library may have access to.

KEY WORDS AND PHRASES

If you are using PICO or SPIDER to look at your question, this will be easy because the key words will come from each part of the framework. However, you should consider any synonyms (these are other words that mean the same thing as the one you are investigating; for example, if you are looking at 'paramedics' you could also include 'emergency medical technicians') to make sure you get the most complete selection.

DATABASE THESAURUS

Some databases have an inbuilt thesaurus which lists the preferred search terms of the database. It can suggest related search terms and broader and narrower terms. If this is the case, try using them. If you have the time and are really keen to get it right, try practicing before you get your first assignment (trust me, it will save time in the long run).

TRUNCATION AND WILDCARDS

These can help you find articles that contain words that are variants of your keywords.

Truncation means applying asterisks to the root of a word, which is the word in its shortest form. For example, using 'dance' as the root word, you would write dance*, which will also search 'dancing', 'dances', 'dancer'…let's be honest, most healthcare professionals like a little boogie from time to time.

Sometimes truncation is not helpful because it can give you too wide a selection of words. If this occurs, consider trying a wildcard, which means inserting a symbol in the middle of a word to find words with a variant spelling. For example, p#diatric finds pediatric or paediatric. The symbol varies depending on which database you are using, so ask your librarian or alternate the following symbols until you select the right one for the database you are using: # or ? or *.

BOOLEAN OPERATORS: PUTTING TERMS TOGETHER

Boolean operators allow you to combine, include and exclude search terms. It sounds complicated, but it isn't; in fact, we already did it a bit earlier on in the chapter.

It is simply using *and*, *or* and *not*. Below is a description of which each does:

- *and* combines two terms together to make a search more specific. Using this will mean that you only find articles which contain both terms. For example, 'paramedics *and* end of life care' would only give you results if both the terms are in the paper.
- *or* helps you find articles which contain either one or both terms. This is useful when there is more than one term for what you are searching for; for example, 'end of life care *or* palliative care'.
- *not* is used to exclude a term from your search to make it more precise. For example, 'paramedics *not* emergency medical technicians' would only show articles containing information about paramedics.

You can use a combination of Boolean operators (*and/or/not*) to create a precise search. For example: 'healthcare professionals *or* paramedics *and* end of life care *or* palliative care *not* general practitioners *not* doctors'.

NARROWING DOWN YOUR SEARCH

It is likely that, even after having carried out a really focused search, you will still have more articles than you know what to do with. It can be tempting to just pick a random one, but that won't look good in your assignment. You need to make it clear how you got from the number of articles you identified in your search to the ones that you have chosen. What you can do now is have a look at the articles, read the abstracts and see if they are actually relevant. You will probably have a few articles that have come up more than once, so you can remove the duplicate ones. Then see if the remaining articles meet your

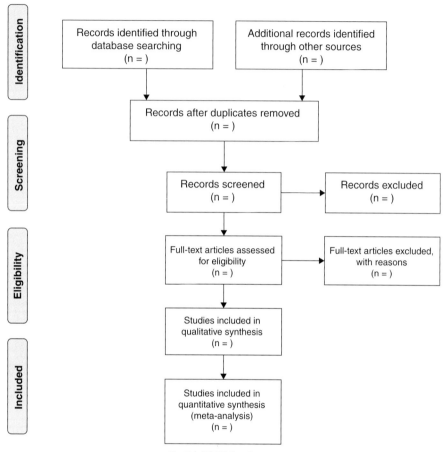

Fig. 5.4 PRISMA flow diagram.

search criteria. To explain how you got the articles that you did, you can use a flow diagram like the one above from the Preferred Reporting Items for Systematic Reviews and Meta-Analyses flow diagram (Moher et al. 2009; Fig. 5.4).

CRITIQUING TOOLS

Critiquing tools are frameworks which give you a set of questions to help you evaluate the worth of a piece of research. It is important to choose the right tool for the job, as some frameworks have questions that are better suited to different types of research, and you would not want to evaluate a qualitative article with a framework that was only designed for quantitative research (or vice versa). As you progress through from level 4 to graduation your lecturer will ask more of you within your work. One of these expectations will be for you to start showing critical analysis skills, and this can include analysis of the evidence you have provided—especially in your dissertation or service improvement module. Getting used to using these frameworks early on will help you in the long run. Here are some of the critiquing frameworks that are most likely to be of use to you as a student paramedic. We have included the names and computer links for you to download them and use them directly—just make sure you add them to your reference list.

- **Critical Appraisals Skills Programme (CASP) Checklists:** This is a mix of eight different frameworks, each covering a different area; for example, systematic reviews, case studies and randomized controlled trials (RCTs). Helpfully, these eight frameworks are also free to download, so no issues there. If you use them for your dissertation you can include them in the appendix, just make sure you reference the source within your reference list. We're not going to tell you much more about them, as they are self-explanatory and really easy to use. The checklists can be found at: https://casp-uk.net/casp-tools-checklists/.

- **Oxford Centre for Evidence-Based Medicine:** This is similar to the CASP checklist, and includes systematic reviews, RCTs, qualitative studies and more. Best advice: look at all the frameworks and pick your favourite. These tools can be found at: https://www.cebm.net/2014/06/critical-appraisal/2.
- **DISCERN:** This is an online and printable framework that can also be used by patients who are deciding treatments, so it is multidimensional. The instrument can be found at: http://www.discern.org.uk/about.php.

Remember: the research might be of good quality, but if it does not apply to you or the subject, then do not use it just for the sake of it.

Literature searching and critiquing is all a matter of practice: the more you do, the better you will get.

REFERENCES

Benger, J.R., Kirby, K., Black, S., et al. (2018). Effect of a strategy of a supraglottic airway device vs tracheal intubation during out-of-hospital cardiac arrest on functional outcome: The AIRWAYS-2 randomized clinical trial. *Journal of the American Medical Association 320*(8):779-791.

Centre for Reviews and Dissemination. (2008). Systematic reviews: CRD's guidance for undertaking reviews in healthcare. York: University of York. Available at: https://www.york.ac.uk/media/crd/Systematic_Reviews.pdf. Accessed on 14/06/2020.

Cooke, A., Smith, D., & Booth, A. (2012). Beyond PICO: The SPIDER tool for qualitative evidence synthesis. *Qualitative Health Research, 22*(10), 1435-1443.

Glover, J., Izzo, D., Odato, K., et al. (2006). *EBM Pyramid.* California: Dartmouth University/Yale University. Available at: https://guides.lib.uci.edu/ebm/pyramid. Accessed on 02/09/2021.

Greenhalgh, T. (2019). *How to read a paper: The basics of evidence based medicine* (6th ed). London: Wiley Blackwell.

Howick, J., Chalmers, I., Glasziou, P., et al. Explanation of the 2011 Oxford Centre for Evidence-Based Medicine (OCEBM) Levels of evidence (background document). Oxford Centre for Evidence-Based Medicine. Available at: http://www.cebm.net/index.aspx?o=5653.

Howick, J., Chalmers, I., Glasziou, P., et al. The 2011 Oxford CEBM Evidence levels of evidence (introductory document). Oxford Centre for Evidence-Based Medicine. Available at: http://www.cebm.net/index.aspx?o=5653.

Moher, D., Liberati, A., Tetzlaff, J., et al. (2009). Preferred reporting items for systematic reviews and meta-analyses: The PRISMA statement. *PLoS Medicine,* 6(7), e1000097.

OCEBM Levels of Evidence Working Group. (2011). The Oxford levels of evidence 2. Oxford Centre for Evidence-Based Medicine. Available at: https://www.cebm.net/index.aspx?o=5653. Accessed on 31/07/2020.

Zhang, Z.J., Yu, X.J., Fu, T., et al. (2020). Novel coronavirus infection in newborn babies under 28 days in China. *European Respiratory Journal.*

ESSAY AND REPORT WRITING

THIS CHAPTER WILL:

- Give an overview of how to structure an essay and a report, and what is expected in each section.
- Give you some advice on how to plan your work.
- Present some examples of essays and reports to give you an idea of the sort of writing you will be expected to do at university, including common mistakes students make and how to avoid them.
- Finally, cover proofreading strategies.

UNDERSTANDING YOUR ESSAY QUESTION

The most important aspect of essay writing is answering the question. Everything you write about in the essay needs to help answer the question, otherwise there is no point in putting it in.

Table 6.1 shows key words used in essay questions that tell you what you should be doing in your essay.

Note the different levels of critical analysis expected. Questions with the key words 'describe' or 'explain' will expect a much lower level of critical analysis than questions that ask you to critically discuss.

Critical analysis is looking at the positives and negatives of a particular subject, fully investigating all the different areas it involves and looking at it from every angle, not just one viewpoint.

An example of this could be: should CPR be given to every patient in cardiac arrest? Someone might automatically say 'yes' because it gives that person a chance of survival. A critical analysis would look at resources, cost implications, chance of survival, end-of-life care, patients' wishes, relatives' wishes, additional hospital pressures, psychological effects on all parties involved...the list can go on and on, and for each area both the positives and negatives would have to be considered.

PLANNING

You may be the sort of person who can knock out an essay in 2 hours, or it may take you much longer. Whether or not you spent much time planning essays before you went to university, you will need to do some planning now. This is because of the need to include evidence and critical analysis, as discussed in Chapter 5. To do this well you need to do a bit more preparation.

Planning is quite a personal process, so it is worth trying different strategies to see what works for you. One thing that really helps, whichever method you use, is to think about what evidence you are going to use for each paragraph in your essay. This way you know you have enough evidence before you start writing.

Here you can see two examples of students' plans for the same essay. One has used a table to form a more linear plan, and the other is a mind map. All students have their preferred method of planning; some like the pictures or flow of the mind map, while others prefer the detail of the linear approach. It does not matter—if it is your first time, then try them both to see which you like most.

MIND MAPS

Mind maps can be good to use if you have a lot of ideas but are not sure what sort of order to put them in (Fig. 6.1).

Table 6.1 Key Terms in Essay Questions

Describe	Outline the main features of something.
Discuss	Using evidence, discuss the positive and negative aspects of the topic in question and come up with your own conclusion.
Evaluate	Consider the strengths and weaknesses of something, or weigh up different options. Come to a conclusion based on the evidence.
Review	Give an overview of what we know about a topic. This should be critical, not descriptive.
Analyse	Look at something methodically in detail so that you can explain and interpret it fully.

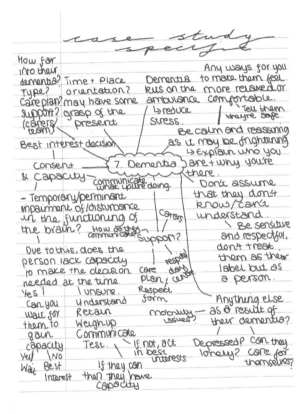

Fig. 6.1 Mind map.

Steps to making a mind map:
1. Start with a central idea in the middle of the page. In this case we have used an ethics essay. You could use the essay title because it might focus you more.
2. Think of as many ideas as you can for things that you can write about in your essay; these are branches of your central idea (key words).
3. Add points related to these as subbranches.
4. You can add details and images to your map.
5. Make connections.

It does not have to be complicated; it just needs to have the five key elements discussed. It is all about getting down the information you need to put in your essay.

LINEAR PLANNING

A simple table (e.g., Table 6.2) can make this easier, and you can build on it when you actually start writing.

MAKING YOUR ESSAY FLOW

You can use the Point-Evidence-Explanation-Link (PEEL) paragraph structure (Fig. 6.2) to make your writing flow and help you with your planning. If you are not sure what would be the best order to put your ideas in, try writing a sentence about the point of each paragraph. Then you can think about how the points link to each other.

Table 6.2 Essay Planning	
Essay title	This will be given to you. If not, look at the question and change it to a title. • Analyse the need for ethics in healthcare—why can't HCPs just follow the law?
Introduction	This is where you tell the reader exactly what you are going to cover in the essay (sometimes this can be written last) and make sure you link it to your learning outcomes. • Within healthcare, ethics are vitally important in the care of… • Within this essay there will be a analysis of the four bioethical principles • This will include…
Main body point 1 Point 2 Point 3 Point 4 Point 5 Point 6	Within each of these sections, put in your key points for discussion. You can also put in key arguments as you progress. Include reference links, and so on. This can be a working document and can develop as needed as you find more information to include. The Point-Evidence-Explanation-Link system (described later) will help.
Summary/ conclusion	This is a summary. As you fill up the points, you can begin to populate this box with brief notes of key points. • Ethics is very subjective, depending on the professional • There are four bioethical principles • The Bolam test can be considered to be…

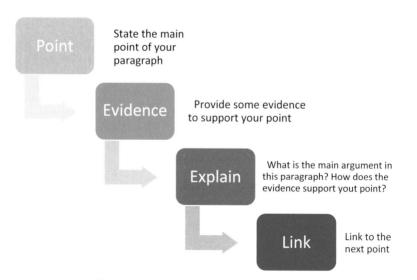

Fig. 6.2 The Point-Evidence-Explanation-Link (PEEL) paragraphs.

SIGNPOSTING PHRASES

Signposting language is words and phrases that explain where you are going to go in your essay and make connections between ideas. You should use signposting language in your introduction and throughout your essay

Signposting in an introduction
This essay will discuss/considers/looks at…
Firstly,…. Secondly,…
Subsequently
Following this…

Signposting to introduce a new point
When looking at…consideration needs to be given to…
…can be identified as pertinent when discussing…

Signposting to introduce a contrasting point or new section
Nevertheless,…
In contrast…

Signposting in the conclusion
In conclusion…/In summary…
Based on the arguments presented in this essay it is clear that…
All this points to the conclusion that…

It is important to think about what connection you want to make between the ideas and choose your words precisely. For example, you should only use 'however' if you are going to introduce a contrasting argument. Try not to overuse these terms.

The Manchester Academic Phrase Bank has more examples of signposting language. It is organized by structure or by function, and can be found at: http://www.phrasebank.manchester.ac.uk/.

So far, we have looked at planning the essay and signposting phrases to make everything flow. Now we need to write the essay, so let's look at structure.

ESSAY STRUCTURE

Introduction (around 10% of the word count)
- What is the **context**? Provide some background information about the topic
- Define **key terms**
- What is **this essay** about (how have you interpreted the question, and what will you focus on)? If you have been given a choice of what to write about, make it clear what you have chosen
- **Structure**. Introduce the main ideas in the order in which you will cover them

INTRODUCTION

A good introduction gives the reader an idea of how you are going to answer the question. In Chapter 2 we talk about the importance of critical writing, and one way you can demonstrate your critical thinking abilities is in your introduction and conclusion. So, you should use your introduction to show that you have an argument to make. Don't just write a generic introduction such as:

> This essay will discuss the treatment of strokes in prehospital care. It will start with an introduction, then the main section will discuss three different types of treatment, and the essay will then end with a conclusion.

Hopefully, it will be obvious that you should not do this, but you will be surprised at how many students do.

Table 6.3 is an example of what you should aim to include in your introduction. Often you won't know what your structure is going to be until you have written the end. In that case, write your introduction last.

Table 6.3 Introduction Inclusions	
In 2019, 1770 people died or were seriously injured on the roads (GOV.UK 2018).	What is the CONTEXT?
Numerous studies have investigated prehospital treatment, which is treatment provided before the patient getting to definitive care, of victims of road traffic accidents. Definitive care can be described as that provided at a major trauma centre. A major trauma centre is a designated hospital fully equipped to deal with major trauma. There are 27 major trauma centres throughout England (NHS 2016).	What do KEY TERMS mean?
This essay discusses multiple treatment options that ambulance crews have when treating major trauma.	WHAT is the essay about?
It does so by introducing major trauma and defining what it is, then exploring three specialist treatment options in turn. This essay will then look at any research in relation to the specific option and will analyse the effectiveness of these three key treatment options, which are...	HOW will this be done? (What is the STRUCTURE?)

The Main Body of the Essay

> **Main Body (around 85% of the word count)**
> - Use a chain of paragraphs to EXPLORE AND DEVELOP YOUR IDEAS/ARGUMENT
> - You will probably have four or five main topics or themes
> - Consider what your main themes are:
>   - Sometimes these are given to you in an assignment brief
>   - They may emerge from your reading or thinking (consider your mind map)
> - Each topic or theme is explored in one or more paragraphs
> - Consider the breakdown of the word count. For example, if each paragraph is 100–200 words, then each theme could be discussed in 500 words, three paragraphs, etc.
> - You can use the Point-Evidence-Explanation-Link tool to structure your paragraphs

Here is an example of the section of the main body of the essay with two connecting paragraphs.

> Tranexamic acid (TXA) is a drug that has been used in major trauma since the 2010 CRASH 2 trial results were published, resulting in a change from 0% of patients receiving the drug in 2010 to 10% in 2016 (Coats et al. 2019). Evidence has identified that if TXA is given within 3 hours of the initial injury to patients who have undergone a major trauma, such as those involved in a RTC, the patients' risk of mortality decreases. An important point to note is that this trial also identified that if TXA is administered outside of the 3-hour window the mortality rate increases (NICE 2012).
>
> One study has shown that patients who are given TXA outside of the 3-hour timeframe are also at a higher risk of emboli, including pulmonary embolism and DVT (Glover et al. 2019), alongside the previously identified risk of death. Therefore, the conclusion can be drawn that...

The Conclusion

We now need to look at the final part of the essay: the conclusion (Table 6.4).

> **Conclusion (around 5% of the word count)**
> Do not introduce any new material here (if it is important, it needs to be included in the main body of the essay).
> - Summarize your main argument. **How have you answered the question?**
> - Why are your conclusions important or **significant**? Are there any wider implications?

Table 6.6 illustrates an example conclusion.

Table 6.4 Sample Conclusion

This essay has demonstrated that there are multiple treatment options available to paramedics when treating major trauma.	Restate the ARGUMENT/ purpose of the essay
The three options discussed are the use of tranexamic acid,…. It has been identified that each treatment option carries both risks and benefits to the patients, and opinions are divided on each of the options…. By equipping clinicians with knowledge of these risks and benefits, they are more likely to be able to alleviate these risks and will also be able to gain informed consent from patients as they can share the full information with them. Clinicians, once informed fully about the treatment options, are more likely to safely implement them in their future practice.	Significance/wider implications

REPORTS

Reports are divided into lots of different sections, each one beginning on a new page. The format of the report that you are being asked to write may differ from the generic structure below, so you should check your assignment brief carefully to make sure you have included everything you need to include. See Table 6.5.

It is important that you get the formatting right for your report. This is much easier if you use the headings and subheadings options in the styles section of Microsoft Word. These options can be found on the Home tab (Fig. 6.3).

If you use these styles, then you can create an automatic table of contents which updates as you add to your report. This will save you time when you are putting the report together (Fig. 6.4).

Table 6.5 Reports

Title page	Here you should include the title of your report, and possibly also your name and the title of the module.
Executive summary/ abstract	This should be a one-paragraph summary of your whole report, including the introduction, main sections and conclusion.
Table of contents	List the contents in the order they appear in your report. Use numbered headings and subheadings.
Introduction	Outline key background information about your topic. Why is it important? Set it in the context of previous research. Outline the aims and objectives.
Discussion	This is the main body of your report and will usually be made up of several sections and subsections. Each section should have a subtitle (follow the guidance given in your assignment brief). Make sure that everything you write is supported by evidence, and that you have shown critical analysis.
Conclusions	How have you addressed your report's aims and objectives? What are the most important points you have made?
Recommendations	Based on the findings of the report, what do you recommend? You can use bullet points in this section.
References	Include all the sources you have referred to in the report, referenced according to your course's referencing style.
Appendices	These are documents that add to the reader's understanding of the report but do not need to be in the report itself, such as additional data. They should be numbered and included in the table of contents.

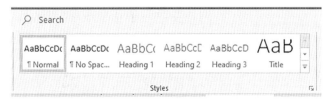

Fig. 6.3 Formating.

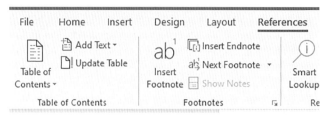

Fig. 6.4 Updating tables.

If you need to include any data in your report, make sure that the table or chart is clearly labelled and has a title. You should also include a reference so readers know where you got the data from.

HELP! MY ESSAY OR REPORT HAS GONE WRONG!

Sometimes, even with the best will in the world, your essay or report doesn't go to plan. It might be that you have gone too far over the word count, you have written lots of bits that don't quite fit together or you have no idea what to write for your conclusion. If this happens, make yourself a cup of tea, sit down and go through the following steps:
1. Have another look at your assignment guidance. Make sure you know exactly what you need to do.
2. Read through what you have written, picking out the key points you want to make.
3. Write a short outline of the main points of your essay. You could use the first sentence of each paragraph; however, if the first sentence of your paragraphs are too long you should write a one-sentence or bullet-pointed summary.
4. Have a look at your outline, then answer the following questions:
   - Are your points in a logical order? If you are not sure, ask someone else to have a look and see if they can follow what you have written.
   - Have you repeated yourself?
   - Is there anything that you need to include that you have missed out? Use the assignment brief for this. Is there anything in there that is not relevant?
   - Does each paragraph have one point? Are some of them too long or too short?
5. Once you have done this, make a new plan, remembering to use the PEEL paragraph structure. Open a new Word document and copy and paste anything that is still relevant. Fill in any gaps, making sure that the first sentence of each paragraph makes it clear what it is about.

PROOFREADING STRATEGIES

Proofreading is an important part of completing your assignment. It can really help with the clarity and presentation of your assignment. If your essay is easy to read, this will make it easy for your lecturer to award you marks. When you are checking your work you might want to have a look at the section on writing with clarity in Chapter 2. These are some strategies that can help you proofread your work:
- Read your work out loud. You can often hear mistakes that you can't see.
- Personalize your proofreading. Get to know the sorts of mistakes you make often, and actively check for them.
- There are some apps that help with proofreading. Grammarly is a free app that plugs into Microsoft Word. It checks for grammar errors and explains what the grammar rules are so you can learn from your mistakes.

Proofreading is extremely important to finish off your essay, and it can be the difference between grade boundaries or even passing or not. Just be aware that universities often have proofreading policies, if you are asking someone else to help you out. Check with your institution to see if they do have one, but an easy rule of thumb is to not ask someone else on your course, as this could lead to issues with possible collusion (working too closely together). Also, make sure your proofreader is just looking to make sure your essay makes sense (if it doesn't, you need to change it) and that the spelling and grammar are correct; they must not correct the content.

REFERENCES

Coats, T.J., Fragoso-Iñiguez, M., & Roberts, I. (2019). Implementation of tranexamic acid for bleeding trauma patients: A longitudinal and cross-sectional study. *Emergency Medicine Journal.* 36,78–81.

Glover, T.E., Sumpter, J.E., Ercole, A., et al. (2019). Pulmonary embolism following complex trauma: UK MTC observational study. *Emergency Medicine Journal.* 36, 608–612.

NHS. (2016). Major trauma centres in England [Online]. Available at: https://www.nhs.uk/NHSEngland/AboutNHSservices/Emergencyandurgentcareservices/Documents/2016/MTS-map.pdf. Accessed on 14/06/2020.

NICE. (2012). Significant haemorrhage following trauma: tranexamic acid [Online]. Available at: https://www.nice.org.uk/advice/esuom1/chapter/key-points-from-the-evidence. Accessed on 04/06/2020.

University of Manchester. (2020). Academic Phrasebank [Online]. Available at: http://www.phrasebank.manchester.ac.uk/. Accessed on 20/04/2020.

EXAMS

CHAPTER OUTLINE

IN THIS CHAPTER, WE WILL COVER:

- Planning your revision.
- Different revision strategies.
- The different types of exams you might have to sit.
- Strategies for the exam.

INTRODUCTION

Exams: love them or hate them (and let's face it, more people are in the hate camp), they are an important part of university life, and no matter what you are studying at some point you will more than likely sit an exam.

Everyone will have their own personal history of taking exams, and it is easy to let that colour your attitude towards them, especially if it has not been a good experience. However, like anything else in life, revision and sitting exams are skills you can learn and develop, so do not worry.

If you consider exams you have previously sat, some of them GCSE or A levels, then these are just stepping stones to this career, which is something you really want and are interested in: this really helps.

If you have had a bad experience (and let's be honest, the bad experience is normally failing—otherwise people tend to forget the 'exam pressures' once they have passed), reflect what your past experience of exams has been and why were they good or bad, if the latter consider why was it a bad experience and is there anything you can do to change it. Consider the following:

- Do you need to alter your frame of mind?
- Do you need to consider strategies to deal with stress?

> Remember, the purpose of an exam is just to test your knowledge. No one who sets an exam wants students to fail: firstly, universities want their students to pass because this demonstrates they are teaching the right stuff; and secondly, if you fail they have to mark your work twice, so they will help you as much as possible. Accept the help and guidance given. This could be revision sessions, online help, question banks, mock exams…the list goes on.

WHAT TYPES OF EXAMS MIGHT YOU HAVE ON A HEALTHCARE PROFESSIONAL DEGREE COURSE?

There are five main types of exams:
- Multiple choice questions
- Calculations (maths)
- Short-answer questions
- Long-answer question
- Seen exam

REVISION STRATEGIES

Start by working out what you need to revise.

Exam revision can feel overwhelming. It is easy to feel swamped by how much you need to revise and worry that you are missing out on something important. That is why it is important to plan out your revision.

If you can, get a copy of a past exam to help you prepare. You should also familiarize yourself with the expectations of the module. Have a look at the module handbook, if you have one, to see what the expectations are:
- Look at the learning outcomes of the module.
- Find out about the format of the exam. What type of questions will it have? If possible, get a copy of a past paper to help you prepare.
- Find out what topics could come up. If anything from your course or module could come up, then you need to map it out (Fig. 7.1).

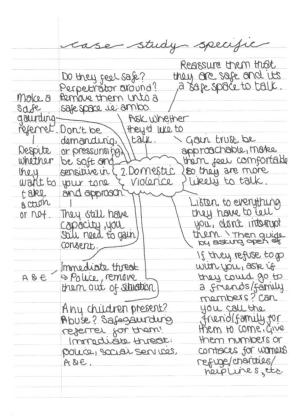

Fig. 7.1 Revision table.

To do this, get a copy of your module handbook and your lecture notes. Make a big mind map of everything that could come up. The reason that a mind map is good for this is that you can link topics together in the branches.

Once you have done this, identify the areas that you are confident about and those that you are not confident about. (In the picture, the areas ticked are the ones the student is confident about.) Try to identify things that are mostly likely to come up. These could be:

- Topics that are covered in the learning outcomes
- Things that are going to be essential to your role as a paramedic or healthcare professional
- Topics that you have covered in lectures or seminars (lecturers often put a lot of emphasis on things that are likely to come up); look at lecture titles or PowerPoint titles

This should give you an idea of everything you should cover in your revision and which topics that you need to focus on.

Also, do not forget the simple solution of asking the lecturer: he or she will often direct you as to what areas to look at.

PLANNING YOUR TIME

Work backwards from your exam date to make a plan of what subjects you need to cover and when. It is important to not focus all your time in one area and leave another key area until there is no time left to revise. You need to make sure you are making good use of your time. Let's be honest, normally there will be a lot more to do in your life than revise, be that lectures, work or family commitments, or just not wanting to spend every spare minute revising, so you have to revise 'smart' (Fig. 7.2).

MEMORY RETENTION—KEEPING IT IN YOUR HEAD

We will be honest, one of our biggest problems is keeping information in our heads. We understand things when we are told them, but then the information just disappears. We have come to the conclusion that it falls out of our ears when we are asleep…or maybe, just maybe, there is some research somewhere that states after 3 days a person only retains 10% to 20% of written or spoken information. However, research also identifies that 65% of the information you have seen (visually) is retained, so when you are revising consider whether you should use just text or audio, or text + audio + visual. Yep, you are much more likely to remember something if you can make it as visual as you can.

CHUNKING

We can hold five chunks of information in short-term memory. However, these chunks can vary a lot in size.

You have probably been using this strategy for years without knowing it. Think of how you remember phone numbers.

MNEMONICS

One strategy that relates to this is using mnemonics. Mnemonics is using a pattern of letters to make something easier to remember.

For example, the mnemonic 'SOCRATES' can be used to find out more about a patient's pain:

- **S**ite
- **O**nset

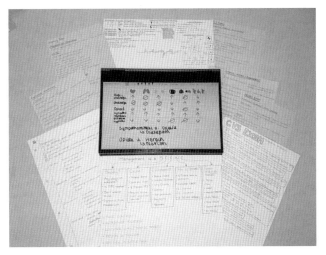

Fig. 7.2 Revision, revision, revision.

- **C**haracter
- **R**adiation
- **A**lleviating factors
- **T**iming
- **E**xacerbating factors
- **S**everity (1–10)

WHEN TO REVISE

This is really subjective and depends on the person and his or her lifestyle; there really is no right or wrong answer. Some people would rather do revision at 0700 in the morning, when they feel fresh and ready for the day, whereas others might rather revise at night when they have peace and quiet. Just remember to try not to revise when you are too tired because the information will do that falling-out-your-ears trick!

LEARNING ANATOMY AND PHYSIOLOGY

One of the subjects that is most likely to come up on an exam in healthcare is anatomy and physiology. There are two types of healthcare professionals: those who just get a subject, and those who have to work on it. We definitely fall into the latter category; that being said, it has to be learned…after all, who wants someone looking after them who does not know their arse from their elbow (hopefully you can write that in a book)?

There are a few ways to revise anatomy and physiology. One of the best ways we have found is using mind maps—yep, not the first time we have mentioned them.

MIND MAPS

Making a mind map is a step-by-step process. You need to make one out for each subject you need to cover; do not try to cover too much in one mind map. You need to break information down into as much detail as you might need for the exam, like the example shown in Fig. 7.1.

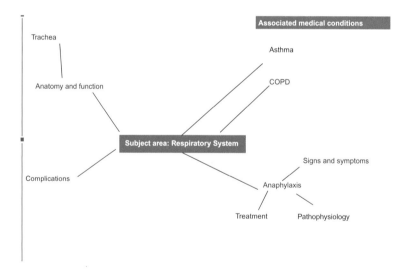

This is just the start of a mind map in relation to the respiratory system; it will help you direct your revision.

A useful revision skill could be to have an original map and then to redraw it with the important information included, and compare the two to make sure you have not missed anything. Remember that you will need to go into detail. You might need to use a general mind map to work out what you need to study, then a different one for each area.

You could make one blank map to fill in for each subject, then you will be used to the framework and less likely to forget information in short-answer questions as you work through your mind map in your head.

There are other ways to revise, although, if mind mapping is not what you like you could try some of the ideas below.

BULLETED LIST WITH HIGHLIGHTS

For example:
- Muscular skeletal system
  - 206 bones in an adult body

- ○ Types of bones
  - Long (femur)
  - Short (metacarpals)
  - Flat (ribs)
  - Irregular (vertebrae)
- ○ Tendons
  - Attach muscle to bone

VISUALIZATION SOFTWARE SUCH AS VISIBLE BODY

There are lots of visualization software packages now that detail the intricacies of the human body, and a lot of these are interactive so you can look in detail at different areas. It is worth asking your librarian if there are any that the university has purchased.

COLOUR CODING

It can help to write different information in different colours. For example, all the general information about a body system can be written in blue, then the conditions associated in red and the signs and symptoms in green…for some people this really works.

ANATOMY AND PHYSIOLOGY COLOURING BOOKS

Quite a few of the publishers have now brought out anatomy and physiology colouring books for students to use. These can really help when you are having to learn things like muscles and bones, but also they have also included things like the anatomy of the heart or the cranial nerves. Once you have completed the colouring books you can use them as visual revision guides.

FLASH CARDS

Flash cards are a great way to learn key facts and make sure you cover all of the topics in your module. Traditionally you would use index cards to make them, but you can now get apps that let you make electronic flashcards and test yourself on your phone or tablet (there are a lot—Google them to find the one that works for you; Cram is one that works on Android and iPhone, for example).

    If you would rather make your own, here are some tips:
- Write questions or key terms to test yourself on one side of the card (one idea, one flash card)
- Put the answer on the reverse side of the card
- Try to guess the answer before turning the card over to check
- Sort your cards into two piles: one pile for the answers you were confident about, and the other pile for those you were unsure of

How many bones are there in the human body?	Adult 206 Children >300

REVIEWING YOUR FLASH CARDS

The best way to review your flash cards is by using a technique called spaced repetition. This is based on research into memory, which shows it is more effective to review the information several times at spaced intervals than it is to revise in one big chunk.

    For example, you could review the information:
- The same day
- 24 hours later
- 3 days later
- 1 week later
- 1 month later

    This means that you are reviewing the information before you forget it.

    Review the cards you were not sure of more regularly than the known cards. If you use flash cards, you can also get others to help you revise: ask them to ask you a question randomly, and then tell them the answer, and if you don't know just revisit it later. Undertaking revision sessions with others in your group can help you (and them) learn as well.

    Flow charts can be another revision tool, similar to bullets and mind maps. You just need to put the information in a flow chart. These can be better for people who like flow and order because mind maps can get messy.

There are other resources available to you such as fill-in-the-blanks sheets—lecturers might give you these, or you and your study partners (if you like revising in groups) could make them up and then get the rest of the group to fill them in. Make sure you have an answer sheet, although, in case you forget! You could just be testing mnemonics or more complex subjects, for example:

Fill in the missing words:

S......... O......... C......... R......... A......... T......... E......... S.........

OR

Fill in the blanks:

The partial pressure for inspired oxygen is .... mmHg.

DIFFERENT TYPES OF EXAMS

It is good to get to know the different types of exam questions that could come up in your exam, as different questions have different expectations. If you are not sure whether a question expects a long, essay-type answer or a short answer, have a look at the way the question is worded and the number of marks available.

Look at the two questions below. Which one is a short answer, and which one would require an essay style answer?
1. Describe how the body regulates blood pressure.
2. Discuss the concept of a duty of care in relation to paramedic practice.

As question 1 asks you to describe, this is looking for a short answer.

Question 2 asks to discuss. It is looking for a more in-depth, critical answer where you consider different perspectives. Have a look at Chapter 2 for guidance on how to answer essay style questions.

SHORT-ANSWER QUESTIONS

This is a straight question which requires a simple answer. You just need to remember facts. The number of marks will tell you how much you need to write. When marking short-answer questions, lecturers will normally have a mark sheet in front of them with a list of key words that you will need to mention to get full marks.

For example, if the question asks you to describe the pathophysiology of anaphylaxis (10 points), the lecturer might be looking for the words:
• Allergen
• IgE
• Mast cells
• Histamines
• Cytokines
• Vasodilation
• Systemic effect
• Immunologically- or nonimmunologically-mediated response
• Bronchospasm
• Hypotension

Be aware this is just an example, in case you get this exam question...

IN THE EXAM

Firstly, work out what you are being asked, and be sure to include only that information—don't just waffle because this will just take up time.

Read the question…Read the question…Read the question

Have I mentioned that you need to read the question? You need to understand it, otherwise you will lose marks. State your points clearly, so each one stands out from the others, and try to make one point (in a single sentence or bullet point) for each mark available.

ESSAY

Exam essays are looking for an analytical and critical response to the question. In this case, it is not just about remembering facts, but showing that you have a considered opinion on the topic.

When revising for essay questions:

- Think of different essay questions that could come up and make a plan for them.
- Consider what the key theories you are learning about are and how can you apply them to the topics you are learning about.
- Practice doing some questions in the time you will have in the actual exam. Once you have done this, you will have an idea of how much you can write in the time allocated. You can use this to change your plans. If you did not have time to write everything you wanted to, then prioritize your points.
  During the exam:
- Read the question and underline the key words
- Make a plan
- Make sure you have a clear introduction and conclusion
- Have clear paragraphs
- Be selective—make the most important points first
- Show the links between ideas
- Be analytical: include the 'hows' and the 'whys' in your answer, not just the 'whats'
- Show your working: don't just make a point, outline how you got to that point, along with your reasons and evidence

MULTIPLE CHOICE

If you have dyslexia or other specific learning differences, exams might really worry you (they did us). There are some tricks you can learn to help that can be used across the board.

MEMORY STRATEGIES

A lot of the revision strategies in the section earlier would be helpful for people with dyslexia. However, you may find that you need to repeat certain topics a bit more for the information to sink in. This is called overlearning, and you need to plan for this in your revision schedule. We never did this in our studies, which may be why the stuff fell out of our ears at night.

EXAM ARRANGEMENTS

All universities should take the fact that you have dyslexia into account when making exam arrangements. This usually includes having extra time, and can also include other arrangements such as being able to use a computer, depending on what your assessment of need says. However, it takes time to put these arrangements into place, and it is up to you to notify the university of your needs and provide appropriate proof. Most universities will have a cutoff time for application for exam arrangements. Make sure you let them know as early as possible so you will be able to get what you need.

What you really need to know if you do have specific learning needs is that there are a lot of people in healthcare that do, and they do really well. It might have slowed you down in the past, and we have heard of some bad experiences, but we can tell you from experience that universities now are really supportive, and if you take the assistance offered to you there really is no need to struggle.

WHAT IS THE MARKER LOOKING FOR?

Not just facts. We have discussed short-answer question key words, but the marker needs to see understanding of the subject as well.

Make sure you provide clear answers. Trust me, there is nothing worse than having to dig around an exam paper trying to find the correct answer. Be clear.

DOING WELL ON THE DAY

Some people will wake up on the morning of the exam bright and breezy and all ready to go, whereas others will not have fallen asleep till late (last-minute cramming—never a good idea), and will be really nervous and telling themselves they are not going to pass.

A lot of how well you do on the exam day is about state of mind. This is often what distinguishes those who do well in exams from those who don't.

It is all about getting into the zone—yep, okay, cheese central, but if you have the right state of mind that is half the battle.

Don't panic: you are going to be a healthcare professional. Remain calm.

If you are starting to feel nervous and a little overwhelmed (yes, it is okay to feel that way or to not feel that way) try focusing on your breathing for a little while, keep it rhythmic, regular and smooth. You could also try listening to some music or doing anything that normally calms you down.

It will help if you make a plan for exam day in advance. Here are some pointers:

- Decide how you will allocate your time in the exam
- If you get the chance to choose questions, identify your best topics

- Take 5 to 10 minutes at the start to read the questions
- Take 10 minutes at the end to check your answers
- Divide your time in proportion to the marks awarded for each question
- Stop once you reach your time limit

- Find out:
  - When and where the exam will take place
  - The length of the exam
  - The number of questions
  - The time allowed for the exam
- Practice doing the exam to time; this can help develop your writing speed
- Check key points such as parking and travel time
- Eat before going in
- And yes, use the loo: there is nothing worse than needing to go midexam (who can bet a nervous wee?)

EXAM INFO SHEET

Often universities will publish an exam information sheet, which could be exam-specific or could be a generic one on the university website. These sheets include rules about what you can take in with you and what the instructions are for the exams. Look for them, as you do not want to fail because of an administrative (on your side) error; for example, not leaving enough travel time.

CHAPTER 8

OBJECTIVE STRUCTURED CLINICAL EXAMINATIONS/OBJECTIVE STRUCTURED PRACTICAL EXAMINATIONS AND VIVA VOCE EXAMINATIONS

IN THIS CHAPTER, WE WILL DISCUSS:

- What objective structured clinical examinations and objective structured practical examinations are.
- What to expect on the day.
- What to do to pass.
- An example objective structured clinical examination marking sheet.
- The different levels needed to 'get the higher grades'.
- Viva voce examinations.

The next area that we need to look at is objective structured clinical examinations (OSCEs)/objective structured practical examination (OSPEs) and viva voces. Don't panic if you haven't got any of these on your course—some courses do, and some do not.

Remember that the makeup of any university course is undertaken by the team at the university, and then it goes through an internal validation process and, in some cases (such as any course that leads to registration), an external validation process. This process includes the governing body of the course, for example the HCPC. As long as the courses cover all the content set out by the governing and associated bodies, how the course is run and what learning outcomes are assessed are up to the individual university.

So let's look at OSCE and OSPE exams first.

OSCE stands for 'objective structured clinical examination', and OPSE stands for 'objective structured practical examination'. So what is the difference between the two? The answer is nothing: it just depends on which university you go to as what it is called. Just for ease when writing we will refer to OSCEs in the text, but rest assured we are talking about both.

OBJECTIVE STRUCTURED CLINICAL EXAMINATIONS AND OBJECTIVE STRUCTURED PRACTICAL EXAMINATIONS

These exams are designed to test the practical application of what you have learned; in other words, whether you can undertake the clinical skills of a paramedic or healthcare professional in a practical situation. OSCEs can cause lots of worry or be very stressful. This is dependent on the student. Some worry they will not be able to undertake and remember the skill under pressure, whereas others might feel embarrassed undertaking the examination with people watching. Yet others might love this type of assessment.

Quite often there will be multiple stations to complete during the exam, and these can last from 10 minutes through to an hour, depending on the complexity of what is being assessed. For example, if you are being assessed on a specific system such as the respiratory system, then this exam might only last 15 minutes. However, if you are being assessed on a major trauma scenario, it is more likely to last an hour—which makes sense really because there is more to do!

There are a few benefits of these types of assessment. Firstly and most importantly there is normally a preset marking structure that is made available for students. This means that if you know the structure there will not be any nasty surprises, and you can practice, practice practice until you know every element.

OSCEs are also all about what you can do, rather than what information you can recall. This is really positive when you are going into a practical profession; after all, they assess skills that you will be using every day once you are qualified, unlike written exams.

So How Do They Work?

We could spend ages discussing the OSCEs we have run, but having also undertaken quite a few ourselves while getting my registrations we have come to the conclusion that each OSCE setup is dependent on the university you attend. There are, however, some key similarities:

- You will be asked to register or book in and then show your identification at the start of each OSCE—Do not forget it
- You will be briefed at the start of the OCSE
- You will then be directed to your first station
- Once you have entered you will be told what the station is, either verbally or via a written briefing sheet
- You will be asked to undertake the OSCE, and a timer will be set
- Once you have completed the task and the time has run out you will be thanked and asked to leave
- You will not receive feedback on the day
- It will be run really formally, even if it is being run by your regular lecturers
- Everyone will receive identical briefings for the same situations
- You will be recorded (most likely), or there will be two assessors in the room (this is to ensure that the results are fair and to eliminate any bias)
- Most of the time your 'patient' will be a real person

What To Do To Pass!

- Firstly, remember these are the skills you will be using on a daily basis, so if you tend to panic, don't!
- Make sure you attend all the sessions. This may seem like a silly comment, but your lecturer will go over everything you need to do in the sessions, so if you do not attend then you are really only going to be disadvantaging yourself.
- Get hold of and print off the marking sheet—this will tell you exactly what you need to do to pass the OSCE.
- Look through the sheets and find the 'easy marks'. OCSE sheets often have identical key components. For example, the first mark might be 'introduce yourself to the patient', and the second might be 'gain consent from the patient'. These may well be on each OSCE sheet, so if you ensure you learn these, then you already have two ticks, and ticks equal points. Enough points mean a pass!

OSCEs are like exams in a lot of ways, so make sure you have a look at Chapter 2 which covers areas like how to revise and how to plan revision. These tips and skills can be transferable to OSCE planning and revision. There are also a pass criteria for OSCEs just like for exams, so you need to find out how the points are awarded. For example, if you do the bare basics can you pass, or are there other elements such as interaction with patients or general manner that will award you points for interpersonal skills (some universities will award points for these, and some won't—you need to check)?

MARKING CRITERIA

We have mentioned the marking criteria (Table 8.1), but it will definitely help for you to see an example if you are reading this in advance (unlikely, we know, but hey, there are some super-organized people out there).

WHAT DOES IT ALL MEAN?

If you are presented with an OSCE sheet like this, you need to understand exactly what you need to do to get that important tick in the column that will give you 5 points. Each lecturer will have his or her own point of view, but here is an example for you to work from if you are not sure.

Consider the peripheral examination section:

- If you miss it out you will score a 0.
- If you undertake a few of the peripheral examination tests, such as examining the nails for clubbing, testing for fine tremors or checking the patient's hands for temperature, but do not communicate what you are doing you might get 1 point.
- If you tell the patient (and examiner) you are checking for fine tremors, clubbing and the patient's temperature you might get 2 points.

Table 8.1 Sample Marking Criteria

ASSESSMENT CRITERIA	FAIL (0)	40-49 (1)	50-59 (2)	60-69 (3)	70-79 (4)	80+ (5)
Introduce yourself to the patient						
Gain informed consent*						
Ensure the patient is in the correct position						
Examine patient's environment						
General patient observation: visual						
Peripheral examination						
Head and neck examination						
Inspect: Anterior and posterior*						
Palpate: Anterior and posterior*						
Percuss: Anterior and posterior*						
Auscultate: Anterior and posterior*						
Other specific respiratory system tests						
Handover: ASH-ICE format						

- If you undertake all the tests but do not explain them you will get 3 points.
- To get 4 points you need to explain the tests and say what you are looking for. For example: 'I am checking your fingers for clubbing. If this is present, it can indicate the presence of an underlying health condition such as lung cancer or bronchiectasis'.
- Finally, to get that elusive 5 points you will have to go into even more detail. For example: 'I am now going to check for asterixis. Some people also call this flapping tremors. It is a type of negative myoclonus which can be characterized by irregular lapses of posture causing a flapping motion of the hands. It is caused by carbon dioxide retention which can occur in conditions such as COPD. Other causes of asterixis include hepatic disease and azotemia, which is a build up of nitrogenous products' (Agarwal & Baid 2016).

As you can see, you will need to work hard to get top marks; but if you really understand your subject and practice, you can achieve a lot.

> Do not just learn everything by rote (do not just learn your lines), actually understand what you are saying: then there is less of a chance of freezing in the middle of your objective structured clinical examination.

*CRITICAL FAILS

As you can see by the little* on the OCSE sheet, some universities have things called 'critical fails'. This is dependent on the university, but you do need to look out for them or ask when you are given the OSCE sheets if there are any critical fails. These critical fails can mean that if you forget one of the starred sections you will automatically fail the OSCE, irrespective of your overall score.

> Remember that you can often forget one or two areas (that are not critical fails) and still get enough points to pass the assessment. So if you realize you forgot something after you leave, try not to panic.

PREPARATION

As for any practical assessment or exam you need to prepare yourself and know your stuff.

There are two stages to your preparations for OSCE and viva voce exams, which we are going to discuss later in the chapter. You might read that practice is the key, and in a lot of respects it is, but there is a stage before that, and that is understanding.

Once you understand everything that you are doing and why you are doing it you are less likely to freeze in the exam or get yourself confused. Some people can learn the 'script' and regurgitate it during the OSCE, getting full marks. However, there are two considerations when trying to learn to pass rather than having full understanding. Firstly, if you suddenly forget your lines it is harder to move on to the next element. Secondly, and probably most importantly (and even though this is a study skills book), you are not learning the assessment to pass an exam: you are learning it to do a job—a really important job. If you do not understand it in an exam you will not understand it on the road, so there is no purpose in undertaking the exam.

So now we have got an understanding, the next thing is practice, practice and then practice some more. You can do this in multiple ways. First of all, you might want to practice on your own to build up your confidence. We used sofa cushions made to look like a person and worked through the OSCE in slow time, checking the sheet as we went.

If you are already fairly confident, then you can move on to a 'real' patient. This can be anyone you are comfortable with, be it a classmate, a family member or a friend. What is really important is that you treat practice sessions like the real thing where possible, because, if you add your own little bits of typical healthcare humour into the practice sessions, there is a slim chance they will come out in the real sessions!

Once you are confident with your one-to-one practice then you need a third person, ideally someone with the same medical knowledge as yourself who can be your marker. If you haven't got someone like this, then an option is film yourself doing the OSCE and then mark yourself on it. This can be uncomfortable to start with for some people, but is a really good way of identifying any mistakes or seeing what you have missed out.

EQUIPMENT

For some OSCEs you will be expected to use medical equipment or paramedic bags. You need to have a look at these beforehand and make sure you know where everything is. Just think what would happen if you had a life-support OSCE and spent the first 2 minutes frantically looking through every bag for the bag valve mask: not the best start, and the delay could cause a fail because of what could be considered unsafe practice. If there is other medical equipment that might be used, then make sure you know how it works, and practice with it. Most universities will demonstrate any equipment you are unsure of if you ask—it might be that you learnt how to use it the previous year and have not touched or seen it since.

A little secret: no university wants their students to fail, for multiple reasons. For one, they don't want to have to run more OSCE sessions; and for another, lecturers are really pleased if everyone passes because it means they have taught the students well.

> If in doubt about anything, ask.

VIVA VOCE

The literal meaning to this is 'by voice' (although we're sure it is written in a more eloquent way than in other literature—we go with understandable!).

This means it is an exam, but you speak the answers rather than write them—let's be honest, some people's nightmare and others' joy!

Vivas, as they can be known, can range in time depending on what is being assessed. Because of changing times in education, these vivas are being used more and more within degrees, whereas up until recently they were predominantly used further up the education chain for doctorates and presenting a thesis. Not all allied health courses will include vivas, unlike OSCE, which will be included in the majority of programs.

WHAT CAN BE ASKED?

Within healthcare degrees, vivas are normally structured. This means they are made up of a series of questions that each student will be asked in order. They will also be planned in advance like any written exam, meaning that there will also be a series of answers to go alongside the questions. So you can consider vivas to be similar to exams, and therefore you need to think how you would revise for an exam.

Some examples could be to describe the blood flow through the heart or to point out the different anatomical locations on a model (a human or a skeleton).

HOW THEY WORK

This, like the OSCEs, is dependent on the university. Generally, the starting format is the same as an OSCE: you will book in and be put in a holding room. You will then be briefed, either as a group or individually as you start the viva. This will give you instructions.

The viva will then happen in front of either one or two assessors. If there is only one assessor it is highly likely it will be videoed. This is because the external examiner will need to review the video to make sure the marks are correct and that everyone has been treated fairly. The video can also be used to recap marks and to identify any problems (or not) if the student complains about his or her mark.

Note that an external examiner is a completely independent person, normally from another university, who looks over all the assessments to make sure that the assessments are fair before they are issued and that the marking of the assessments is fair.

REVISION

More often than not if you have a series of multiple choice questions on an exam paper, you may work in pairs or study groups, asking each other verbal questions. This technique will help you revise and prepare for a viva. It will build up your confidence in listening to questions and then answering them verbally. Some people prefer to read the questions, so being verbally asked questions within an exam might be a completely different experience; the more you practice, the easier you will find it.

EQUIPMENT

Sometimes in vivas you might be given props or information sheets. For example, you may have a person or a skeleton to use to identify anatomical landmarks.

If you do have a model you need to make sure that you are clear when you are pointing to an anatomical location and do not just point in a vague area. This is a way you can fail without even realizing it. You might be given numerous anatomical models—just ensure that, if possible, you have a look at them beforehand and identify all the landmarks yourself, as during the viva it is likely you will be given a time limit to answer the questions.

COMMUNICATION

As a clinician you need to make sure that your communication is very good. After all, you are going to have to speak to patients all the time. If you haven't had a lot of experience speaking to strangers, you could consider working with someone on your course who you wouldn't normally work with or asking a friend of a friend to ask you questions or be your patient for an OSCE run through. This seems silly, but the more you do it the more comfortable you will feel with people you do not know.

Communication also needs to be clear. If you mumble the answer to a question or mumble when you are undertaking the OSCE, then the examiner will not know what you are saying. This could lead you to not being awarded points for information that you have actually covered, which could be the difference between passing or not: a shame if you actually know your stuff.

Hints and tips for objective structured clinical examinations and vivas:
- Find out what is being tested and make sure you revise the correct subject.
- Use the time you have been given—try not to rush things. If you have time left over to recap exactly what you have done, you might remember something you have missed out.
- Dress professionally in either a neat and tidy uniform or smart but practical clothing. Tie long hair up and, for the practical lesson, make sure you are bare below the elbow (NHS guidance).
- Listen to the question or read any information sheets carefully—make sure you know what is being asked of you.
- Be confident in what you are saying or in the procedure or skill you are undertaking. The examiner will have more confidence in your ability if you do not dither.
- Consider your attitude and deportment—manners and a friendly attitude will go a long way.
- Listen to your patient and what he or she is saying—recap what he or she has told you. This will show both the patient and the examiner that you have been listening, and might stop you missing an important clue.
- If you do not understand a question or an information sheet, then ask the examiner—you will waste time and marks if you answer the wrong question or undertake the wrong exam.
- Practice. If practice sessions or mocks are offered, make sure you attend and take every opportunity to get your hands on patients or simulate situations.

AND FINALLY, NERVES

Throughout this whole book we have talked about different exams and assessments, but one area we have not really covered is nerves. These could be nerves about exams, OSCEs, viva voce assessments, writing your first assignment or undertaking your first presentation. Nerves can sneak in when you least expect them. Remember that being nervous is okay. No really, it is okay! Generally, being nervous means you are passionate about the subject—although you can be passionate without nerves (don't worry), a few nerves are good. It is only when the nerves become overwhelming that they become an issue. If this happens, take a moment to tell yourself 'this is okay', take some deep breaths and remind yourself that you know your stuff and that if you forget something it is not the end of the world. You will have committed the starting few points to memory, so start with them—or if you don't know the answer to a question, think about it; then, if you still don't know the answer, move on: it is okay not to know everything, and you might remember it later.

REFERENCE

Agarwal, R., & Baid, R. (2016). Asterixis. *Journal of Postgraduate Medicine, 62*(2),115-117.

PRESENTATIONS AND ACADEMIC POSTERS

IN THIS CHAPTER, WE WILL COVER:

- Presentations
- Planning and preparation
- Using visual aids
- Success on the day
- Academic posters
- Poster design
- Research
- Content
- Presenting

During your course you might be required to undertake presentations at different points. These will be across a range of areas, and you might be asked to do presentations as part of your seminar after undertaking some research. Alternatively, you might be asked to undertake a presentation as a formative assessment. These are informal assessments that normally work towards a summative assessment and that you will get marked on. Summative presentations might actually form part of your course as well; these might be standalone presentations or presentation of your academic poster. We will discuss these later; right now we are going to focus on general presentations.

PLANNING YOUR PRESENTATION

The secret to doing a good presentation is to plan well. Ok, so it's not that much of a secret, but if you prepare well you will do well, even if you are not a natural public speaker.

There are lots of different structures you can follow. Below we describe how we tend to plan our presentations by breaking the process down into stages.

Stage one: Before you start preparing your presentation (Table 9.1).

You will need to know the answers to all the questions above before you consider starting to write/plan/prepare (whatever you want to call it!) your presentation.

Let's break stage one in a little more detail.

Aims and objectives: Consider looking at the learning outcomes (if it is an assignment). Are there key elements you need to include? For example, if you are discussing the need to do an ankle x-ray, then do you need to include signs and symptoms or national guidelines such as National Institute for Health and Care Excellence guidelines?

Who is the presentation actually aimed at? This is really important because it will tell you the amount of detail you need to go into and how to 'pitch' your presentation. If you are giving it to mentors, then you know you need to go into a lot of detail, and you can assume a certain level of knowledge. If you have been asked to present to your peers about a new subject, you will have to explain the basics and then build up to the more in-depth knowledge.

Where are you presenting? Although this might not affect the content of the presentation, it will affect how you present. Think about it: if you are in a big lecturer theatre that holds 150 people, you are going to have to project your voice, and often (not always) you could be more nervous; so considering how much time you have until the presentation, you might want to factor in a practice. If you are in a classroom you might be able to change the seating around to suit you—you would have to check on this though.

Table 9.1 Stage 1

Aims and objectives	You need to consider what you are trying to achieve in the presentation (well, in addition to passing, obviously!).
Who is the presentation actually for or aimed at?	For example, are you presenting information to the rest of your group/lecturers, or to an external person (e.g., your mentors from placement or your placement providers; it could be anyone)?
Where are you presenting?	Often this will be in a classroom, but we have seen presentations take place in large lecturer theatres.
Technical bits	How long have you got/will you have the use of information technology/have you been given any guidance on style or font size if you are using slides (if slides are allowed), and so on.

The technical bits: Before you plan any presentation you need to understand the guidance you have been given. The first thing you should consider is how long your presentation needs to be. Most presentations you will be asked to give at university are short, and you don't want to overload your talk. If you are using computer slides to help you with your presentation, then the general rule of thumb is one slide for every 2 minutes you have to talk. For example, a 10-minute presentation will contain five slides, or a 20-minute presentation 10 slides—this excludes the reference slides.

If you decide to research this further, there are lots of figures for introduction timings and questions and answer times, but if you work from the 2-minutes-per-slide rule you won't go far wrong.

As with all the assessments we have discussed, make sure you actually understand the timings. For example, you may have been asked to undertake a 10-minute presentation with a further 5 minutes at the end to answer questions. If you're not told, then ask!

You can lose marks automatically if you deviate from the guidance (if you have any) on font size or length of presentation. Often in formal assessments you will be stopped at the end of the allotted time, so if you don't plan well, then you might not have time to cover one of the key learning points.

People often think that there will automatically be information technology (IT) available for them to use, but this is not always the case. If there is IT, then how will you upload your slides? Consider whether can you use a memory stick, or if will you need to email the presentation in advance; you might be asked to upload it to Turnitin (the system universities use to check you have not copied each other or just cut and pasted).

Stage 2: Preparing your presentation (Table 9.2).

Key points: If you are giving an assessed presentation, have a look at the assessment criteria and make sure you cover everything that you need to. We have said this on numerous occasions, but look at the assessment guidance and see what you are being asked to do—get that trusty highlighter pen out and highlight the key areas. Check, check and recheck you have covered everything—there is no point waffling on about treating pain levels in fractures for 90% of the presentation if the actual learning outcome is to identify and explain the guidelines in relation to the diagnosis and treatment of a fracture—you simply will not pass.

Pick a platform: If you are able to use IT in support of your presentation, there are a few programs you can use. Probably the most popular is PowerPoint, which allows you to design a range of slides to present with. You can also do things like embed videos, use animation, add images, include different fonts and animations—and a whole lot more. There are numerous other platforms though; you just need to check if the university system supports them, or that you can attach your laptop to the big screen.

Other options are;

Table 9.2 Stage 2

Key points	What must you discuss in your presentation to cover the aims and objectives.
Pick a platform	There are multiple platforms, such as PowerPoint or Prezi. Alternatively, you might just wish to talk and not use any supporting platform.
Structure your presentation	There are numerous elements to a presentation. You need to plan what information will go where; actually using a presentation grid or a mind map will help.
Find the supporting evidence	Because it is a presentation-style assessment at university, you will be expected to use a variety of high-quality supporting evidence.
Critical writing and thinking	Again, like providing supporting evidence, you need to follow the academic style of thinking and writing and ensure that you present at the academic levels we discussed in the academic writing chapter.

- **Google slides:** This is a free part of the basic Google account package. It is similar to PowerPoint and can be accessed as long as you have access to the internet (you need to consider the strength of signal). It can also be updated in real time, so if you share it with the group, for example, and want to add something more after the presentation, you can update it and the link will automatically update— you do not have to resend like PowerPoint.
- **Prezi:** This is the platform used when presenters wish to share their presentations on the internet with the general population. One of the things that Prezi does that PowerPoint and Google Slides does not is show the whole presentation at once and then allow you to zoom in to different sections. This makes Prezi ideal for slightly less formal presentations (ask your lecturer if they are happy to have a Prezi presentation used for a formal presentation if you would like to use it; it can make yours standout).

PowerPoint, Google Slides and Prezi are just three possible presentation platforms. There are multiple others that have not been mentioned.

Good practice:
- Use a large font: 26 points or bigger
- Use easy-to-read fonts: Arial or Verdana are the most widely used
- Choose a professional font (nothing too curvy, which can be hard to read)
- Use dark text on a light background
- Use the slides to support your presentation, not be your presentation

Bad practice:
- Using lashing or unreadable colour combinations
- Overusing special effects such as zoom or spins
- Making overloaded slides

STRUCTURING YOUR PRESENTATION

Within any presentation there need to be certain elements: an introduction (the beginning), a main body (the middle bit) and a summary (the end!). Let's apply this to the previous example of 'identify and explain the guidelines in relation to the diagnosis and treatment of a fracture' (Table 9.3):

Table 9.3 Structure

	Introduce yourself and the title of your presentation, then state the key areas you are going to discuss in the main body of the presentation, such as: • signs and symptoms of a fracture • the national guidelines for x-ray • the treatment of a fracture
Main body: Break it down into clear sections linked to the main ideas.	In this example you would use the key area as headings—one on each slide, with a summary. You would then talk in more depth about each subject. You can use academic references within the verbal part of your presentation. For example, on the slide you could have: • Diagnosis of an ankle fracture - NICE guideline - Ottawa ankle (NICE 2016) You would then explain the Ottawa ankle rules to the audience in more detail.

Summary: Briefly sum up your main points. Nothing new should be introduced; this is where you recap the learning objectives.	This is a summary of the key points you have covered. Do not go into detail because you have already done this.
	For example:
	• Multiple tools for the diagnosis of fractures
	   ○ Ottawa ankle rules
	   ○ Physical examination
	   ○ Visual examination
	   ○ History
	• Treatment
	   ○ Immobilization
	   ○ Pain relief
	   ○ ...You get the idea.

Reference slide: This is excluded from the 2 minutes-per-slide rule.	It is highly likely you will need a slide of references at the end (don't read this out; it is just for information).

SUPPORTING EVIDENCE

Critical writing and thinking: Everything we have said in this book about critical thinking in academic writing also applies to presentations (check out the chapter if you are not sure what we're talking about). Ask yourself: why am I telling my audience this? How do the points that I am making in the presentation link together? Is this information part of the learning objectives, additional useful information in support or just waffle to fill the time? Often presentations are short, and you have a lot of information to give to the audience, so make sure the information you are providing meets the aims of your presentation.

When you are researching, keep track of all the sources you use. Remember that you need to include references in your slides. If you use charts or pictures, you need to reference them too.

PRESENTING CONFIDENTLY

Almost everyone feels some degree of nerves when it comes to public speaking. It really is one of those things where the more you do it the easier it gets. If you are worried about doing a presentation, then make sure you practice beforehand. Get to know your content well enough that you can talk without reading off the slides.

If the presentation is assessed, it is worth practicing doing it on time. Then you will know if you have the right amount of content. It is best to try and speak a bit slower than you normally do so that the audience has the chance to take in what you are saying. Consider how you stand.

Make sure you have your PowerPoint saved in at least two different ways: the last thing you want to do is to lose your USB stick. If you have your presentation saved somewhere in the cloud (such as One Drive), you are not going to lose it forever.

DEALING WITH NERVES

A big part of successful presentations is body language. If you smile and make eye contact with the audience, this will make a good impression. If you are nervous, just pick one person in the audience to look at.

BE PROFESSIONAL

You need to consider professionalism before you even walk into the room. Consider how you are dressed: ripped jeans and a sweatshirt do not portray the image of a healthcare professional. Some lecturers will expect you to have made an effort, and it can also help with your confidence—sometimes that smart attire can be like wearing a uniform, and this can help look the part/feel the part!

You need to consider your language as well: swearing or using slang words will not show you in your best light, and some universities have 'portraying a professional image' as part of the marking criteria.

Finally, arrive in plenty of time. Running in just before the doors are closed will not put you in the right frame of mind. Also, if you are not there by the start time then it is unlikely (like an exam) that you will be let into the room.

MARKING CRITERIA

As for any academic piece of work, there will be a marking criteria. We have mentioned this regarding a professional image, but there are lots of other potential areas in which to gain (or loose) marks. So make sure you look at the marking criteria and cover everything in them. For example, the assessor could be looking at the following criteria:
- Relevance to practice
- Presentation skills
- Covering the learning outcomes
- Professional image
- Quality of supporting presentation

Each area could hold a different rating; for example, each could be 20 points to make 100%, or learning outcomes could be worth 40 points, with 15 points assigned to each of the other areas. I think we have said it before: Ask!

ACADEMIC POSTERS

Academic posters are not the normal posters you have probably been asked to produce up to now—that is, if this is your first university experience. They are academic pieces of work that have certain elements and requirements, and they can take as long to produce as an essay or assignment because they include full academic research and require referencing.

Academic posters are often used at conferences as an easy way of sharing findings and presenting information. You might be asked to undertake research or investigate one particular area and present your findings. A good poster uses a combination of visual elements and text to get your point across. Sometimes you will be asked to do a presentation based on your poster (a poster presentation); if this is the case, you will have to put a lot of work into both.

PLANNING YOUR POSTER

Before you start planning, check your assessment requirements. These are some of the things you should consider:
- Who is the poster audience? A poster aimed at healthcare professionals will be different to one aimed at the general public.
- Is there a word limit?
- What size does your poster need to be?

It is important to be selective about content. You can't fit everything on your poster. You should aim for three main points, plus an introduction and conclusion. It is a good idea to use images and graphs to try to convey some of the information. You still need to write in an academic style and use formal language and references. It is ok to use bullet points (which you should avoid if you are writing an essay).

LAYOUT

Consider the order that you want people to read your poster in. Make sure your points are in a logical order. We read from left to right, so that is a better order. Put the most important information in bold and use larger font sizes so readers can identify the main points.

You can make posters using a range of different software programs. The ones that are easiest to use are PowerPoint and Microsoft Publisher.

In PowerPoint use the slide size feature on the design tab to change the slide to the correct size for the poster.

Here is a good example of an information academic poster (permission was kindly granted by the author) (Fig. 9.1). The other option is a research poster Fig. 9.2.

KEY TIPS

- You must include references in your poster.
- Consider the background of your poster: You must make sure that it does not detract from what you have written, (i.e., make sure you can see the writing and that it stands out). If you are not sure, ask a someone to look for you and see if they can read it easily.
- Consider using diagrams to highlight points—just remember that diagrams, images and text need to be referenced if they came from an external source.
- Plan your poster like you would a presentation or an essay: get a piece of paper and section it off with what you are going to put in each area.
- Don't forget, it is an academic piece of work.

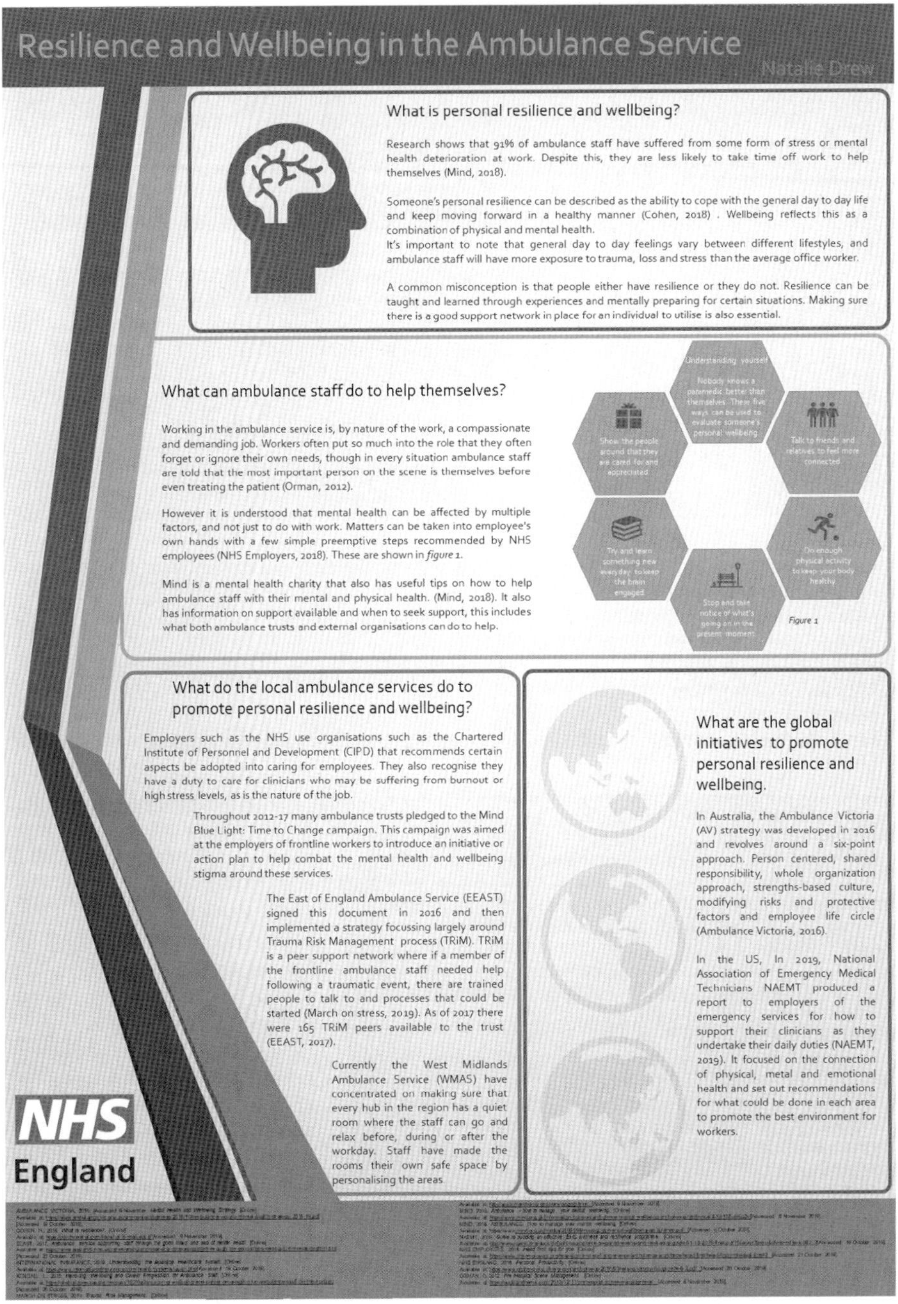
Resilience and Wellbeing in the Ambulance Service
Natalie Drew
What is personal resilience and wellbeing?
Research shows that 91% of ambulance staff have suffered from some form of stress or mental health deterioration at work. Despite this, they are less likely to take time off work to help themselves (Mind, 2018).
Someone's personal resilience can be described as the ability to cope with the general day to day life and keep moving forward in a healthy manner (Cohen, 2018) . Wellbeing reflects this as a combination of physical and mental health.
It's important to note that general day to day feelings vary between different lifestyles, and ambulance staff will have more exposure to trauma, loss and stress than the average office worker.
A common misconception is that people either have resilience or they do not. Resilience can be taught and learned through experiences and mentally preparing for certain situations. Making sure there is a good support network in place for an individual to utilise is also essential.
What can ambulance staff do to help themselves?
Working in the ambulance service is, by nature of the work, a compassionate and demanding job. Workers often put so much into the role that they often forget or ignore their own needs, though in every situation ambulance staff are told that the most important person on the scene is themselves before even treating the patient (Orman, 2012).
However it is understood that mental health can be affected by multiple factors, and not just to do with work. Matters can be taken into employee's own hands with a few simple preemptive steps recommended by NHS employees (NHS Employers, 2018). These are shown in figure 1.
Mind is a mental health charity that also has useful tips on how to help ambulance staff with their mental and physical health. (Mind, 2018). It also has information on support available and when to seek support, this includes what both ambulance trusts and external organisations can do to help.
Understanding yourself
Nobody knows a paramedic better than themselves. These five ways can be used to evaluate someone's personal wellbeing
Show the people around that they are cared for and appreciated
Talk to friends and relatives to feel more connected
Try and learn something new everyday to keep the brain engaged
Do enough physical activity to keep your body healthy
Stop and take notice of what's going on in the present moment
Figure 1
What do the local ambulance services do to promote personal resilience and wellbeing?
Employers such as the NHS use organisations such as the Chartered Institute of Personnel and Development (CIPD) that recommends certain aspects be adopted into caring for employees. They also recognise they have a duty to care for clinicians who may be suffering from burnout or high stress levels, as is the nature of the job.
Throughout 2012-17 many ambulance trusts pledged to the Mind Blue Light: Time to Change campaign. This campaign was aimed at the employers of frontline workers to introduce an initiative or action plan to help combat the mental health and wellbeing stigma around these services.
The East of England Ambulance Service (EEAST) signed this document in 2016 and then implemented a strategy focussing largely around Trauma Risk Management process (TRiM). TRiM is a peer support network where if a member of the frontline ambulance staff needed help following a traumatic event, there are trained people to talk to and processes that could be started (March on stress, 2019). As of 2017 there were 165 TRiM peers available to the trust (EEAST, 2017).
Currently the West Midlands Ambulance Service (WMAS) have concentrated on making sure that every hub in the region has a quiet room where the staff can go and relax before, during or after the workday. Staff have made the rooms their own safe space by personalising the areas.
What are the global initiatives to promote personal resilience and wellbeing.
In Australia, the Ambulance Victoria (AV) strategy was developed in 2016 and revolves around a six-point approach. Person centered, shared responsibility, whole organization approach, strengths-based culture, modifying risks and protective factors and employee life circle (Ambulance Victoria, 2016).
In the US, In 2019, National Association of Emergency Medical Technicians NAEMT produced a report to employers of the emergency services for how to support their clinicians as they undertake their daily duties (NAEMT, 2019). It focused on the connection of physical, metal and emotional health and set out recommendations for what could be done in each area to promote the best environment for workers.
NHS
England

Fig. 9.1 Academic information poster

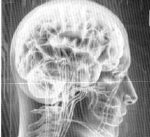

Transient Ischaemic Attack 999 Emergency Referral feasibility trial (TIER): Recruitment and intervention usage

C Hampton[1], N Rees [2], J Bulger[1], K Ali[3], T Quinn[4], G Ford[5], A Akbari[1], M Ward[6], A Porter[1], C Jones[2], H Snooks[1]
[1] Swansea University, [2] Welsh Ambulance Service Trust (WAST), [3] Brighton and Sussex Medical School, [4] Kingston University and Saint George's University, [5] Oxford Academic Health Science Network, [6] West Midlands Ambulance Service

Background

Early specialist assessment of Transient Ischaemic Attack (TIA) can reduce the risk of stroke and death. This study assessed feasibility of undertaking a multi-centre randomised trial to evaluate clinical and cost effectiveness of referral of patients attended by emergency ambulance Paramedic with low-risk TIA directly to specialist TIA clinic for early review.

Methods

- Developed a protocol and referral pathway for Paramedics to assess patients
- Paramedics who volunteered to participate were randomly allocated to intervention or control group
- Intervention Paramedics were trained to deliver the intervention during the patient recruitment period
- Control paramedics continued to deliver care as usual
- Patients with TIA were identified from hospital records
- We aimed to recruit 86 patients over a 12 month recruitment period and pre-defined progression criteria related to feasibility of intervention delivery and trial methods.

Results

-Development and recruitment phases are complete with outcome follow up ongoing
-89 of 134 (66%) paramedics participated in TIER
-53 (3.8%) of 1377 patients identified as having a TIA from hospital records during the patient recruitment period were attended by a TIER Paramedic and identified as eligible for trial inclusion
-3 of 36 (8%) patients attended by intervention paramedics were referred directly to the TIA clinic
-1 incident appeared to be a eligible for referral but attended the ED
-1 was attended by an Intervention paramedic who was not TIER trained
-1 patient record was missing
-1 patient was refused a TIA Clinic referral and was referred to their own GP
-All others attended by intervention Paramedics (n=29) were recorded with contraindications to receiving referral: FAST positive (n=13); ABCD2 score >3 (n=5); already taking warfarin (n=2); crescendo TIA (n=1) other clinical factors (n=8)

- Preliminary results indicate challenges in recruitment and low referral rates.
- The low-risk 999 TIA population suitable for Emergency Department avoidance may be smaller than previously thought.
- Further analyses will focus on whether progression criteria for a definitive trial were met, and clinical outcomes from this feasibility trial

This project is funded by Health and Care Research Wales (project number 1053). The views and opinions expressed are those of the authors and do not necessarily reflect those of Health and Care Research Wales, NHS Wales or Welsh Government.

Fig. 9.2 Academic research poster

REFERENCES

NICE. (2016). Fractures (non-complex): assessment and management [Online]. Available at: https://www.nice.org.uk/guidance/NG38/chapter/Recommendations#acute-stage-assessment-and-diagnostic-imaging. Accessed on 31/07/2020.
http://www.primecentre.wales/resources/TIER%20Int%20Dev%20and%20Usage%20Poster_2018.pdf

REFLECTIVE PRACTICES

IN THIS CHAPTER WE WILL:

- Discuss why reflective practice is so important as a paramedic.
- Look at some of the different models of reflection you can use, including the National Health Service structured reflection template, Gibb's reflective cycle and Willis's reflective models for paramedics.
- Provide an example of a piece of reflective writing.
- Finally, give some advice on how to use evidence in your reflections.

Often when placements are involved within a course, reflective practice is required. This reflection does not cease when leaving university: it can continue through your professional career. Therefore, getting it right straight away is imperative.

The Health Care Professional Council (HCPC, 2019) states:

> 'Reflective practice allows an individual to continually improve the quality of care they provide and gives multidisciplinary teams the opportunity to reflect and discuss openly and honestly.'

The HCPC is the regulating body for allied health professionals—not an organization to ignore. If you would like to know more about the HCPC, their website is: https://www.hcpc-uk.org/ (Fig. 10.1).

So what do some students really think about reflective practice: that it is something to be gotten through, a waste of time, a hoop they have to jump through to pass, boring…? The list can go on and on, and we'll be honest; when we were students, we thought most of those things.

Next you need to consider what professionals think about reflective practice. Well, let me set the scene with an ambulance case study (something one of the authors experienced, incidentally, when she was a trainee; clearly with all identifiable information removed).

The team responded to a call to an 85-year-old patient with a fever who was on chemotherapy for cancer. Clinically it was clear that the patient was unwell, with a high temperature, fast heart rate and lowering blood pressure, and was clammy to the touch—all clear signs of what can be called a 'big sick' patient. So the patient was transported to the nearest A&E and kept in the queue. Once it was their turn to hand over to the much more experienced (and a little scary) nurse, the nurse listened intently to the handover and immediately exclaimed: 'Why didn't you prealert us (that is the term for letting them know in advance) that this patient needs isolation? She might have neutropenic sepsis, put her in side room 2.' (Just a side note: this was before the Surviving Sepsis Campaign, for those of you who are wondering about a time when sepsis wasn't really thought about in prehospital care.)

The author did as she was bid and then walked off, not understanding exactly what she had done wrong. So off she went and spoke to her mentor, who told her to do a reflection on the job and then come back and ask again. That's what she did, and she didn't need to go back to her mentor because by undertaking a reflection she realized exactly what she had done wrong and what effects that could have had on her patient. In the 15 years since the reflection she has never forgotten what neutropenic sepsis is and the precautions needed for this patient group.

So remember: reflection is done when the student or professional has something to reflect on. It is designed to help you look at a specific job or event and then assess if it could have been undertaken in a better way or to strengthen knowledge for the next time you come across it.

Remember that reflections do not have to just be clinical. You could reflect on your communication at an incident or how you lead a team; reflections are for anything that you think you would like to improve on or to consider what you have done. They can also be used if you feel unsure about a job (consider a major trauma or multiple patient incident). Reflections can be done for anything.

Reflect on things you are not sure about or that have concerned you so that you can learn from them. This will stop you from the feeling of it being a waste of time; it is really where you can make changes in your practice. It also allows you to show development to your tutors and demonstrates continuing professional development (CPD) to the HCPC.

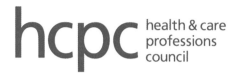

Fig. 10.1 HCPC

REFLECTION MODELS

There are lots of reflective models/frameworks that you can use, and each university lecturer and clinical practitioner will have his or her favourite. Check with the university to ensure that they do not have a specific model they would like you to use. If they do not mind, then you could pick one of the models below or research others until you find one you like.

Box 10.1 shows the NHS England Structured Reflective Template. (https://www.england.nhs.uk/south/wp-content/uploads/sites/6/2017/07/cpd-structured-reflective-template.pdf) Box 10.2 shows the Gibbs Reflective Cycle.

The Gibbs reflective cycle (Gibbs 1988) has been used by many practitioners, and it can be used in prehospital care. Using the Gibbs framework can be both an advantage and disadvantage, as it does discuss feelings, which can be good when reflecting on jobs that have caused an emotional reaction; however, if you are looking at jobs that do not involve feelings and emotions, then it can seem a bit long-winded.

Willis's (2010) models of reflection are fairly new to the scene. He has identified that one type of reflection does not always fit each individual job. He has therefore designed three different models that depend on the type of incident you are reflecting on (Fig. 10.2).

All three models encourage you to learn from evidence, which makes your reflections contemporary (Willis 2010) (Fig.10.3).

Here is a list of the models and the most appropriate situations to use them in:

1. Model 1 is used in a situation that you want to learn from by gathering information with a focus on the ethical aspect of care.
2. Model 2 reflects on the human factors that may have had an impact on patient care, such as team working (Fig. 10.4).

Box 10.1 Structured Reflective Template

Name of practitioner: Write in your name.

Registering body number: This could be your Health Care Professional Council registration number or Nursing and Midwifery Council/General Medical Council registration number—obviously this is for when you are qualified; if you are still a student, leave it blank.

Date of incident: Ensure the date will not reveal any personal data; if it was a massive car accident or something that was reported on, then just put a year in.

Description of incident: Stick to the clinical facts, (e.g., 85-year-old female presenting clinically unwell, temp 39.3); do not include any personal, identifiable details.

Overview of reflections/learning from the experience: This is how you felt and what learning came from this reflection—why are you reflecting on this particular job?

You can also use this section to demonstrate learning; just make sure you reference anything that comes from literature, as detailed in Chapter 3.

So you could write, for example:

The National Institute for Health and Care Excellence (2019) states that, in a patient that has risk factors for neutropenia such as current chemotherapy, neutropenic sepsis must be suspected.

Describe how this learning will be put into practice: This is what you plan to do in the future—how would you change things if you feel you could improve on your practice.

Any further action/learning identified: You might have identified that you would like more training within a specific area, or you might like to undertake some research. If you do not feel any further action or learning is needed, then put 'not applicable'; but remember, it could just be as simple as reviewing current guidelines regularly.

Box 10.2 Gibbs Reflective Cycle

Description: What happened in the job.

Feelings: What were you feeling before and after the incident.

Evaluation: What was good or bad about the experience.

Analysis: What sense can you make of the incident—why did you do what you did, and what were the challenges?

Conclusion: What have you learnt (consider looking at literature here)?

Action plan: What would you do if you came across this situation again?

Description - What happened in the job	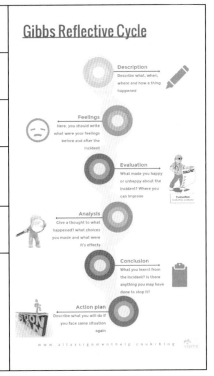
Feelings - What were you feeling before and after the incident	
Evaluation - What was good or bad about the experience	
Analysis - What sense can you make of the incident - why did you do what you did & what were the challenges	
Conclusion - What have you learnt (consider looking at literature here)	
Action plan - what would you do if you came across this situation again	

Fig. 10.2 Gibbs Reflective Cycle

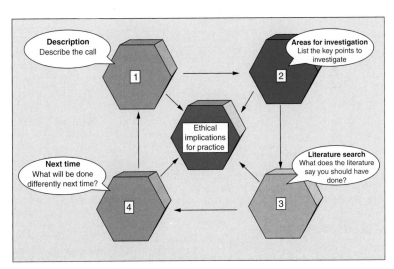

Fig. 10.3 Gathering information (From Willis (2010))

3. Model 3 encourages you to investigate different referral pathways for your patient (Fig 10.5).

It really does not matter what reflective framework you use, unless you have been directed by your university to use one specific one. They are all very similar to one another, and it is all about getting the information down on paper and actually improving your practice.

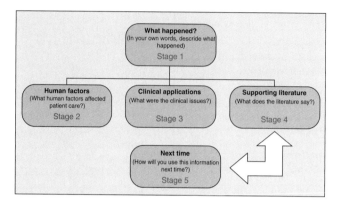

Fig. 10.4 Human Factors (From Willis (2010))

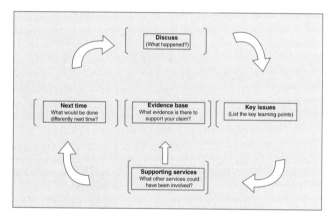

Fig. 10.5 Referal pathways (From Willis (2010))

Reflection allows you to show development to your tutors and demonstrate CPD to the HCPC, which is vital for registration. Each year some paramedics and other allied health professionals will be selected for audit by the HCPC, and these reflections can demonstrate your CPD, which will allow you to maintain your registration.

WRITING YOUR REFLECTION

As you can see from the models, there are a lot of different things you need to include in your reflection. The most important of these is to demonstrate what you actually learned: that is all a reflection is. It helps guide you when reflecting, gives you a focus and allows you to show off what you know.

This sounds really obvious, but a common mistake people tend to make with reflection is to write far too much in the description part. This only tells the reader what is needed to understand why you have reflected: think about it as an introduction that sets the scene, rather than as the main section.

The good thing about reflective writing is that you can (usually) write in the first person (I did, I think that...). This can make it easier to write; however, you do still need to include references in your reflection (see Chapter 3).

What your lecturers and the HCPC are looking for is to link the evidence to what you have learned: in other words, you can not just make it up!

You do not need to be too descriptive here. For example:

The Joint Royal Colleges Ambulance Liaison Committee (2019) states that one of the '6 Ps' of ischaemia is paralysis, so when patient X presented with loss of movement in his left arm, I needed to rule out the causes of ischaemia and check for the other five Ps, these being…instead of automatically presuming the patient had had a stroke.

FINDING EVIDENCE TO USE IN YOUR REFLECTION

If you are not sure what sort of evidence might be useful for your reflection, here are some things to consider:

- **How does your experience relate to HCPC professional standards?** These are the standards of conduct, performance and ethics; your specific standards of proficiency (your particular job specialism, i.e., paramedic); standards of continuing professional development; and standards relevant to education and training. If you are unsure of any of these the most current standards are available on the HCPC website: https://www.hcpc-uk.org/standards/.
- **Your trust policies.** Each individual trust has variations in policies that can cover a wide variety of topics, from how to check your equipment to procedures you must follow when treating a patient.
- **NICE guidelines.** These are guidelines on how to treat and manage your patient's condition. They constitute national advice and are generic throughout the health care system. The most recent information can be found on the NICE website: https://www.nice.org.uk/About/What-we-do/Our-Programmes/NICE-guidance/NICE-guidelines.
- **Any relevant legislation.** Legislation means laws that must be followed in relation to your patient. These laws can cover multiple areas, (e.g., the Mental Health Act), which you might use if you are reflecting on patient consent and capacity. All legislation can be found at: https://www.gov.uk/.

All professional standards such as NICE guidelines, HCPC guidance and trust policies are reviewed regularly; therefore you need to ensure you go straight to the main source and avoid websites that might be outdated.

So let's have a look at an example. We have put it into boxes because this can sometimes help you make sure that you cover everything when you are doing a reflection (you can always remove the boxes after you have finished). Box 10.3 shows Willis's first framework.

Box 10.3 Willis's Model 1

Describe the call

I received a call at 0415 to an 85-year-old female who had fallen and hit her head. On arrival the patient was found sitting on the floor with a hematoma above her right eye with no other apparent injuries. A full history was taken; the pertinent findings being past medical history of AF, diabetes and arthritis which was widespread, treated by Apixaban (2.5mg bd) , metformin (500mg tds) and Paracetamol (1g sos) .

The patient stated she tripped over the carpet and stumbled and fell. She grabbed her bed to break her fall but hit her head on the frame. She also stated she wasn't knocked out or felt dizzy at any time and had no other symptoms.

During a full neuro assessment there were NAD (no abnormalities detected). The only apparent injury was a small hematoma above her right eye with no neurological impairment and the patient stating no pain. The patient was assisted to her feet and she walked with her frame as normal to her armchair and stated thank you very much she didn't wish to attend hospital and she would sign whatever was needed, refusing to go.

I knew that the patient needed to attend hospital, but she refused even after I told her all the risks of staying at home. As an NQP (newly qualified paramedic) I called the support desk, and they spoke to the patient. After they spoke to her, they said it was okay to leave her at home but to let her GP know what had happened.

After the incident I was confused because I felt she should have gone to hospital and leaving her at home was dangerous for her; she might have a bleed to the brain and died. I told her but she still refused. I was expecting the support desk to tell her she had to go but they didn't.

Areas for investigation: List the key points to investigate

1. What are the possible complications of a head injury?
2. What does the advice say in regards to going to hospital with a head injury?
3. Was it ethical to leave her at home with an injury that could worsen with no one to look after her?
4. Why did the support desk say she could stay at home?

Literature search: What does the literature say you should have done?

1. The NHS (2018) states that there can be multiple complications with a head injury; these can be concussion, impaired consciousness, brain injury amongst other complications.
2. Most head injuries are not serious and do not need hospital treatment unless the patient fits into a criteria, one of these being if the patient takes anticoagulant (e.g., warfarin). This patient is on apixaban. This is an anticoagulant and as per NHS guidance (2018) the patient should have received further care at hospital. This is further supported by NICE guidelines in which it states a patient with a head injury who is on anticoagulants should receive a CT scan within 8 hours of the initial injury.

Continued on following page

Box 10.3 Willis's Model 1 (*Continued*)

3. When looking at ethics then, the 4 bioethical principles need to be considered, Eaton (2019) identifies these are nonmaleficence, autonomy, beneficence and justice.

When looking into this case it is autonomy that is key; this is ensuring the patient can make their own decision relating to their care as long as they have all the available facts. Consent and capacity is also important to ensure they can make informed decisions surround their care. This comes under the Mental Capacity Act 2005. In this case it is clear that after I had undertaken a capacity test that the patient did have full capacity to make her own decisions about her care regardless of the consequences and as long as she had all the relevant information and capacity to make the decision, the decision was hers to make.

4. From looking in to consent and capacity and the bioethical principles it has become evident why the support desk came to the decision they did because it was a decision for the patient to make not me as a crew member. I just needed to offer her all the options and tell the all the information surround her current injury and potential complications. This is also mirrored in the HCPC standards of conduct, performance and ethics (2016) in which it states "You must make sure that you have consent from service users or other appropriate authority before you provide care, treatment or other services".

Next time: What will be done differently next time

Next time I attend a patient I will ensure they have all the facts about their condition including potential complications, advice for treatment and other care pathways available. I will then allow the patient to reach a decision as to their care.

When I speak to the support desk (I have to do this to discharge any patient at home), I will explain all the facts surrounding the patient's illness or injuries. I will also ensure they are informed of my full discussions about consent and capacity and the patients decisions relating to care.

(From Willis, S. (2010). Becoming a reflective practitioner: frameworks for the prehospital professional. J Paramed Pract. 2(5):212 -2016.)

REFERENCES

Eaton, 2019EatonLaw and Ethics for Paramedics2019Class PublishingBridgewater.
Gibbs, 1988GibbsG.Learning by Doing: A guide to teaching and learning methods1988Oxford PolytechnicOxford Further Educational Unit.
HCPC, 2016HCPCStandards of conduct, performance and ethics. Available at: https://www.hcpc-uk.org/standards/standards-of-conduct-performance-and-ethics/2016. Accessed 5 December 2020.
NHS, 2018NHSComplications, severe head injury. Available at: https://www.nhs.uk/conditions/severe-head-injury/complications/2018. Accessed 15 May 2020.
NICE, 2014NICEHead injury, quality standards. Available at: https://www.nice.org.uk/guidance/qs74/chapter/quality-statement-2-ct-head-scans-for-people-taking-anticoagulants2014. Accessed 15 May 2020.
Willis, 2010WillisS.Becoming a reflective practitioner: frameworks for the prehospital professionalJ Paramed Pract.2520102122016.

CASE STUDIES

IN THIS CHAPTER WE WILL:

- Begin by explaining what case studies are and the type of case study assignments that you may have to do.
- Demonstrate how to approach a case study assignment, using an example.

Case studies and simulations are used a lot within modern healthcare education, both in teaching terms and sometimes within assessments, and therefore it is important to discuss them both.

WHAT ARE CASE STUDIES?

Case studies often take the format of written information of either a true-life or made-up event. For example:

'Jackson, a paramedic, and Riley, an emergency care assistant working on an ambulance, attended a 16-year-old male 'George' who lives at home with his parents. George had fallen off his push bike on the way to school, and a passerby had called the ambulance.
On examination, they identified an abrasion on his left elbow with some left wrist pain (3/10) and an abrasion to his left knee. They undertook a full examination and found other abnormalities, and also identified the cause of the accident to be George swerving to avoid a second bike that was messing about. They also identified that he had not hit his head and had remained GCS (GCS) 15 throughout.
The crew cleaned and dressed his grazes and then advised George that he should attend the hospital to ensure there were no fractures to his wrist. George told them he was fine and that if they were finished, he'd like to get to school so he was not late. The crew explained that this course of action was against their medical advice, but George refused transportation.
The crew undertook a full capacity test, and George was found to have capacity. He told the crew again that he was refusing hospital treatment and not to bother speaking to his parents because they were at work and he would text them when he got to school. He then signed the patient report form, as did his 17-year-old friend to witness it. They both thanked the crew and rode off on their bikes. The crew then informed control about the refusal to travel and were cleared to attend the next job.

WHEN ARE CASE STUDIES USED?

Case studies are often used because they can get students to put themselves in the situation and investigate as close to real-life problems or dilemmas as possible. Often the lecturers will use situations that they have been in themselves if they are healthcare professionals, which can add another element of realism to the case studies.

Case studies can be twofold. They can be given to students in support of a lecture. For example, if you had undertaken a lecture on ethics, consent and capacity then you might be given a case study about the specific topic and be asked to research it and then bring your ideas to the next session. Consider the example case study. You might be asked to investigate if the patient 'George' was able to make the decision not to go to hospital because of his age, or were the crew ethically right in not contacting the patient's parents. These questions are subjective, but allow you to investigate key areas with something to work from.

Case studies can be about anything at all, like a description of findings from an examination, and you would then have to reach a diagnosis. For example, you could be given the results from a MSK examination and then you could identify any abnormal features or findingsand then you as a student would need to reseach all the possible diagnosis and justify your answer (use evidence to explain how you have come up with these diagnoses.)

CASE STUDIES WITHIN ESSAY QUESTIONS

We have already discussed short- and long-answer questions in exams within Chapter 7, but now we need to look at case studies within assignments.

Depending on the module you are studying, case studies can be a really effective way of focusing attention on the key points. This is demonstrated with a more detailed version of 'George's' case study later.

> Lecturers often want different things in a case study piece of work, so make sure you check what your lecturer actually needs you to do.

WHAT DO LECTURERS WANT?

This is the question all students ask themselves regularly and the answer is easy: it depends on the lecturer. Helpful, we know.

When it comes to case studies, lecturers normally require you to do one of two things:
1. Write an essay purely discussing the case study. For example:
   Within the case study it has been identified that George requested that his parents not be told about the incident and said that he would inform them later; consideration therefore must be given to the fact that George is 16 and still legally classed as a minor or child (DfE, 2018). However, the crew assessed George's capacity and ascertained that George was able to retain information, and...as per NHS (2019) guidance.
   In this example, the case study in integrated into the information.
2. Discussing the learning outcomes or key points, using the case study to support the answer. For example:
   Within the United Kingdom anyone under the age of 18 is legally classed as a minor (United Nations, 1990). However, when considering the age of consent in under-18s, ambulance personnel have to consider if patients have capacity to make decisions surrounding their treatment as per NHS (2019) guidance. Within the case study, the crew have identified that the patient 'George' has capacity.
   In this example the key information is described without using the case study, and then the author uses the case study to reinforce his or her point.
   It is impossible for us to tell you if your lecturers would like option one or option two—some won't mind either way! As we have said previously, if you are unsure, ask.

WHAT TO INCLUDE

If you are given a case study to use for an essay, consider yourself lucky because it will have been written in a such a way that it gives you all the information you need to include. First look at the learning outcomes of the assignment. If we are looking at George's case study, then the learning outcomes might be:
- Be able to describe informed consent and capacity
- Describe and discuss healthcare regulations regarding the treatment of children and young people under 18

So, there are two main 'jobs' to be undertaken. The first job is to look at the case study and highlight the areas that are relevant to the learning outcomes. The easiest way to do this is to grab a highlighter pen for each of the learning outcomes and simply highlight the relevant sections:

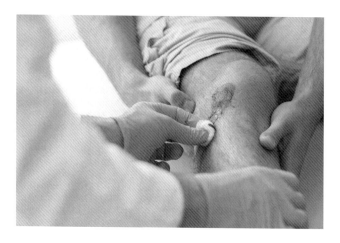

Jackson, a paramedic, and Riley, an emergency care assistant working on an ambulance, attended a 16-year-old male 'George' who lives at home with his parents. George had fallen off his push bike on the way to school, and a passerby had called the ambulance. George tried to tell the passerby not to bother calling an ambulance, but the passerby told him he was too young to make his own decisions and that, because his parents were not there, then an ambulance needed to be called. George tried to argue that he was old enough, but the passerby ignored him.

When the crew arrived, they obtained informed consent and undertook a full medical examination of George. During the physical examination they identified an abrasion on his left elbow with some left wrist pain (3/10) and an abrasion to his left knee. They undertook a full examination and found other abnormalities, and also identified the cause of the accident to be that George had swerved to avoid a second bike that was messing about. They also identified that he had not hit his head and had remained GCS 15 throughout; this was confirmed by witnesses on scene.

The crew cleaned and dressed his grazes and then advised George that he should attend the hospital to ensure there were no fractures to his wrist. George told them he was fine and that if they were finished, he'd like to get to school so he was not late. The crew explained that this course of action was against their medical advice, but George refused transportation.

The crew undertook a two-part full capacity test, and George was found to have capacity. He told the crew again that he was refusing hospital treatment and not to bother speaking to his parents because they were at work and he would text them when he got to school. He then signed the patient report form, as did his 17-year-old friend to witness it. They both thanked the crew and rode off on their bikes. The passerby then approached the crew, clearly unhappy they had let George leave and attend school, saying he did not think it right that they had not taken him to hospital and saying that George was only a child. The crew politely told them that they had fully assessed the situation and the patient in the privacy of the ambulance and thanked the passerby for his assistance. The crew then informed control about the refusal to travel and were cleared to attend the next job.

The second job is to actually research the learning outcomes in this case: what is consent and capacity, and what are the regulations around treating a young person or child? You would need to look at literature, government guidelines, and so on. These need to be looked at in detail and then linked to the case in question.

That being said, occasionally lecturers do just want you to have a look at the case study and tell them what you think clinically. This can work in the same way as already identified: get your highlighter pen out and highlight the relevant areas, think back to the examinations you will have learnt about and identify the findings provided. Make sure you find out what the lecturer actually wants you to do. You might, for example, need to research certain diagnoses or differential diagnoses (other possible causes of the symptoms): remember, there won't just be clues in the physical observations, such as blood pressure or crepitus on movement, you will most likely also be given a history and description of the scene, and all these clues need to be highlighted and then researched (academically if required). If your lecturer does ask you to do this, it will be obvious, and it will be comprehensive if it is an assignment.

You will usually write up your case study in an essay format (see Chapter 2 for more details):

- Introduction
  - Learning outcomes (what the case is about; in the example above it would be about consent and capacity and the legislation around these).
  - You can explain the main points of the case (do not be descriptive here).
- Main body
  - Discuss the main points of the case one by one. You may need to bring in evidence to support each point.
- Conclusion
  - What are the main learning points from the case study?
  - If you have to use references, then you need to produce a full reference list, just like for any other assignment.

REFERENCES

Department for Education. (2018). Working together to safeguard children: a guide to inter-agency working to safeguard and promote the welfare of children. London: Department for Education. Available at: https://assets.publishing.service.gov.uk/government/uploads/system/uploads/attachment_data/file/722305/Working_Together_to_Safeguard_Children_-_Guide.pdf.

NHS. (2019). Assessing Capacity. Available at: https://www.nhs.uk/conditions/consent-to-treatment/capacity/. Accessed 25/03/20.

GROUP WORK

WITHIN THIS CHAPTER:

- First we consider when you might work in groups.
- Then we discuss the factors that make group work successful.
- Next we look at how to organize group work, including written projects.
- After that we discuss how to deal with some of the common problems that you might come across when working in groups.
- Finally, we discuss how to be assertive.

WHEN MIGHT YOU WORK IN GROUPS?

Consider the career path you have chosen to follow: in all aspects of healthcare, people work together in teams and groups. As part of an ambulance crew, consider a cardiac arrest (Fig. 12.1): there is no way a paramedic, nurse, doctor or anyone else can properly undertake full advanced life support without a team around them: http://cardiacscience.co.uk/.

At university you might take part in group work in the following situations:

- Seminars
- Practical simulations
- Group projects
- Presentations

MAKING GROUP WORK WORK

For most people, group work is a positive thing. You get to bounce ideas off other people, and it is more fun than working on your own. However, there are some challenges associated with group work, too, so it is important to think about how to work together effectively. There are three elements to a successful group, as you can see in Fig. 12.2.

Reflection

If you try to make sure that the group has a positive atmosphere and everyone is happy, then it is more likely to be successful. Think of a previous situation where you were in a group that worked well:

- What made the group successful?
- How did you work together?
- What did you bring to the group?

Here is an example of good team working (a team we were part of during a cardiac arrest) that answers each of these questions:

- What made the group (task) successful?
  - Everyone listened to the appointed leader (the paramedic) and took their direction.

- o Each individual knew what he or she needed to do and could competently undertake his or her tasks (e.g., cannulation or chest compressions).
  - o If anyone needed help (like a rest from CPR) he or she asked.
  - o Everyone shared ideas (when discussing moving the patient to the ambulance).
  - o The leader ensured everyone was happy and knew the plan before they did anything.
- How did you work together?
  - o Professionally. Remember that you are on a professional course now (if not already qualified), and are no longer registration students, so for any task you do you need to put aside any differences and bickering and act professional. Differences of opinion are fine, just make sure they are discussed, not argued about. Leave your personal differences at the door.
- What did you bring to the group?
  - o Personally we are paramedics, so we brought those skills to the group, alongside a willingness to listen and take direction.

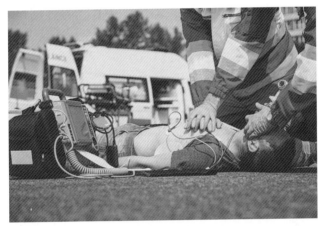

Fig. 12.1 Team work.

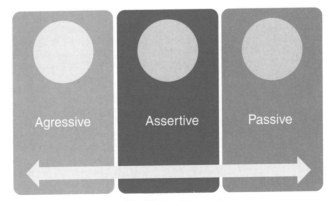

Fig. 12.2 Assertiveness.

GENERAL GUIDANCE AROUND WORKING TOGETHER

It is quite easy to sabotage the group. If you have someone in the group who is always complaining, try to avoid getting sucked into it. Constant complaining does a number of things:
1. It means the person that is constantly complaining gets someone to bounce their issues off.

2. It will bring the rest of the group down and often slow down the work rate.
3. If you join in, it will continue—often people just want to get something out, and once they have, if everyone else is positive, their mood will improve.

Do not be the complainer of the group!

ROLE/TASK ALLOCATION

One thing that can make group work more effective is to allocate roles to each member of the group. For example, in a meeting to discuss undertaking the task, one person could be the note-taker, and one person could be the group chair who is in charge of the discussion and makes sure everyone has the chance to speak.

When you allocate roles to complete the task, no matter what the task might be, it is a good idea to consider everyone's strengths and weaknesses. Consider a cardiac arrest: you wouldn't get a paramedic to undertake chest compressions if a cannula needed inserting and there was an emergency care assistant who was really good at chest compressions sitting there with nothing to do. Remember, you often need to allocate the right person to the right task in healthcare. However, sometimes if the task is not an important one you could also use it as a chance to learn, especially if this is in the university setting rather than at a placement. If you have one person in the group who is really good at presentations, rather than getting him or her to do the whole presentation, try to encourage other less confident members of the group to take a turn to build up their skills. In simulations, often one member of the class will be confident and try to give others the chance to step up. Remember that eventually you will all be professionals in your own right, and you won't have the confident member of your group with you when treating patients. University is a chance to learn and develop, so make the most of every opportunity, even if it is out of your comfort zone.

Some tasks are easier to do as a whole group, such as mind mapping and discussing ideas. Other tasks like researching or writing a first draft are easier to do on your own. Don't think that you have to do everything together.

GETTING ORGANIZED

1. Decide how you are going to work together.
   A lot of groups skip this step because they think it is a waste of time, but it can prevent a lot of problems if you do this. If the task is not a classroom simulation and will take time, then you need to consider various elements. For example, are you going to meet in person or online? Set up some shared folders for your group work using Google Docs or Microsoft Teams. Make sure you have everyone's contact details. It is best to get people's phone numbers as well as email addresses. Find out which is the best way of keeping in touch. This sounds obvious, but it can save a lot of stress.
2. Be clear on the task!
   Have a look at the assessment criteria. Make sure you all understand what you need to do and that everyone in the group has the same understanding of the task.
3. Break it down.
   Think of all the different things you need to do to complete your task. Some things will need to be finished before you can start other things.
4. Create a schedule/plan.
   Work backwards from your deadline and give yourself a bit of a buffer at the end.
5. Allocate tasks and actions effectively.
   A lot of the stress in groups comes from someone feeling they have more work to do than everybody else. It is important to share the task out fairly, not just by giving everyone the same number of tasks, but by making sure you don't lumber one person with a really big task when everyone else gets smaller ones. It is also important to consider the strengths and weaknesses of the members of the group when giving out the tasks. If something turns out to be harder than you anticipated, you can reallocate it.
6. Have regular meetings.
   Keep track of how everyone is getting on, and make sure you are all making progress.
7. Have a back-up plan.
   Sometimes it can be useful to allocate tasks to one main person but also a 'second in command' in case he or she becomes unwell, and so on—this way there is someone who can take over if need be. Information sharing is key to this. This strategy can be put in place for formal presentations. Consider what could happen if only one person has the USB with the presentation on it, or only one person knows the script. At university, this will not be an excuse, and if it is a formal assessment, you will all fail. We have seen the USB excuse numerous times. Trust us when we say it won't wash!
8. Be realistic.
   Be honest about what you can and cannot do. Don't expect too much from other people.
9. Keep people informed.
   Communication is the key to working in groups in any situation.
10. Know when to ask for help.
    If you are struggling with the work, let your group know because they might be able to help you. That's the whole point of working together. If no one knows what to do, go and ask your lecturer.

GROUP DISCUSSION

In groups discussions:
- Include everyone. Try to avoid letting one person dominate the discussion, and if someone is quiet, ask he or she what he or she thinks.
- Listen to other people. Let other people finish before you start talking. Make sure you actually take in what they are saying, don't just sit there waiting to make your point.
- Make use of body language. Think of where you are positioned in relation to other people in the group. Make eye contact and smile.
- Keep everyone on track. Encourage the group to keep to the point, and gently steer them back.
- Disagree in a constructive way. Don't rubbish someone's suggestion. Make a suggestion such as 'have you considered doing it this way' or 'why do you think that…'.
- Build on other people's ideas.
- Contribute, but don't dominate.
- If your idea doesn't get chosen or you don't get the role you want, to put it bluntly, don't sulk: get over it and move on.

WRITTEN ASSIGNMENTS

If you are working on a written assignment such as a group report, the obvious approach is for each group member to take a section of the report and write it individually. However, you will need to put all the sections together and make sure they fit as a coherent whole. Some things to check for include:
- Does the report make sense as a coherent whole?
- Is there any repetition between sections?
- Have you covered everything you need to cover?
- Is it written in the same style? It is not a problem that people write differently, but you want it to be in the same voice (e.g., active or passive) and the same person (first or third).
- Is your use of references consistent? You will need to pull the whole reference list together. This will be the case if you are doing a presentation too.

DEALING WITH PROBLEMS

If you prepare well, you can prevent problems from occurring. Agree how you are going to work together at the start, and you can deal with things better. It is increasingly common now for lecturers to set some kind of self-reflection or peer assessment to be completed after you have done the group work, and sometimes these actually contribute towards your marks. This is because we are wise to the fact that people are more likely to do work if they get marks for it!

Someone Disappears and Hasn't Done Their Share of the Work

This is one of the main things that can go wrong with group work, and it can be a major stress. It is easier to sort out if you have followed the advice discussed and have kept a record of who has been allocated each task, gotten their contact details and designated a second in command. The best thing to try and do is contact him or her (it is good to use email; then you have a trail of evidence that you did contact him or her, so he or she can't turn around and blame you) and say that you are worried that you haven't heard from him or her. Keep him or her informed about your progress and when you are going to meet up so that he or she can come back and rejoin the group.

Make a plan for how you will complete the work if he or she doesn't get back in touch. Even though you have someone who knows about the task, you will still need to reallocate the other person's tasks amongst the group because it would be unfair to ask someone to do two whole tasks by themselves when everyone else is doing one. If you are feeling nice, you could think about what you could give the missing group member to do if they come back at the last minute. Keep your lecturer in the loop. He or she might be able to speak to the group member privately and sort something out. The lecturer could also agree to modify the task a bit so you can hand it in without that person's contribution. Find out if there are any penalties for those who do less.

One Person Does Less

This is a less extreme version of the previous scenario, but the same principles apply. If everyone has agreed what they are going to do at the start, you are within your rights to ask that they do what they are supposed to do. This can be an awkward conversation, but it can be enough to make a difference. These situations are very annoying.

Conflict Between Group Members

Sometimes there can be a personality clash between group members; this isn't unusual and can happen in any team or group. This can cause a lot of tension in the group. If this is not dealt with, it can escalate. It is best to bring this out into the open in a calm way. Give the individuals involved the chance to talk to each other without the other members of the group there. Try to avoid allocating blame. Use some of the assertiveness strategies in the section below.

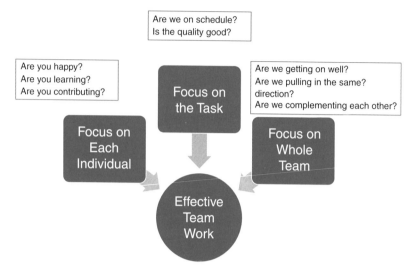

Fig. 12.3 Effective team work.

YOUR GROUP CAN'T AGREE ON WHAT TO DO

If this is the case, give everyone in the group the chance to speak. Listen to their opinions. Write all the suggestions down. If you are not sure of the task, clarify this with the lecturer. It is likely that there are only going to be two or three options that the group can choose between. If this is the case, the best way to decide this is by having an anonymous vote. Once you have chosen what you are going to do, accept this and move on—remember, no sulking!

ASSERTIVENESS

An important skill when working with other people is assertiveness. An assertive person is able to stand up for himself or herself whilst also being respectful of other people. This can be seen as striking a balance between being passive and aggressive (Alberit & Emmons 2017) (Fig. 12.3).

Assertiveness is not:

- **Aggressive:** Assertiveness does not involve forcing people to do things through threats. It does not involve displays of anger (although you may feel angry).
- **Passive:** A passive person doesn't say what his or her own needs are. He or she might 'play the martyr' and let other people get what he or she wants or stay silent when he or she actually wants to speak. Passive behaviour can actually be frustrating for other people because they don't know what you want.
- **Passive aggressive:** Passive aggressive behaviour is when you act passively when it is clear that you are angry. Saying things such as 'do whatever you want' when it is clear you don't mean it, ignoring people or not cooperating are all signs of passive aggressive behaviour. Passive aggressive behaviour can be upsetting to other people and makes situations more difficult to resolve.

> **Reflection**
> Think of someone who is assertive (this could be someone you know; consider the group leaders or teachers you have come across):
> - What makes them assertive?
> - Imagine how they would deal with certain situations.

Pick your battles. A common misconception about assertiveness is that you need to get your own way all the time. This is not the case. Assertiveness is about respecting the rights and needs of both parties in the situation. The ideal is to come to a 'win win' situation. However, because we live in the real world we know that this is not always possible. Sometimes you need to compromise, sometimes you need to concede. Being assertive can take up a lot of energy. If you are in a situation where you can't change the outcome, this might not be a good use of your energy. An assertive person thinks about what is important.

ASSERTIVE COMMUNICATION

An important part of assertive communication is being clear with people about what you actually want. One way of doing this is to use 'I' statements rather than 'you' statements. For example, 'I work better when it is quiet' is more tactful than 'you keep distracting me', and 'I don't agree' is more likely to get a positive response than 'you're wrong'.

An assertive communicator:

- Adopts a calm but firm tone
- Has an open posture
- Makes eye contact
- Is polite
- Does not apologize for asking for something he or she needs

Your tone of voice and body language really do make a difference here. If you are saying something, but your tone of voice implies that your heart isn't really in it, your request may not be effective. If you are not a naturally assertive person, practice in front of the mirror or even with a friend. You may feel silly doing it, but you need to get over any self-consciousness to become more assertive.

One strategy that works when you are trying to get someone to do a specific task is the 'broken record' approach. This means just repeating your point over and over again, no matter how much the person tries to divert you.

CONCLUSION

Working as part of a group or a team can be fun and can really help get a big project completed; plus, you can learn a lot from working with others. Remember that you are going into a profession where working as part of a team is really important. There may well be some disagreements along the way, and it is how you deal with them that could mean a successful project or not.

REFERENCE

Alberti, R. E., & Emmons, M. L. (2017). *Your perfect right: assertiveness and equality in your life and relationships.* 10th ed. Oakland: New Harbinger Publications, Inc.

DISSERTATIONS

IN THIS CHAPTER

- First we outline the different types of dissertations you could be asked to write.
- Then we look at how to choose a topic and title.
- Next we look at how you should structure your dissertation, outlining what you need to put in each section, with some writing examples.
- After that we give you some hints and tips for writing it all up.
- Finally, we have some advice on managing your workload.

For most people, their dissertation is the biggest piece of work that they have done so far, and could even be the longest piece of writing that you will ever do. That sounds scary, but all the assignments you have done at university so far will have helped you to build up to this. You will also be given a dissertation supervisor, a lecturer in your department who is knowledgeable about how to write a dissertation. He or she can give you advice on how to go about investigating your topic, as well as feedback on your writing as you go along.

DIFFERENT TYPES OF DISSERTATION

As we have said many times over the course of this book, different universities have different ways of doing things. This can also apply to dissertations. There are four main dissertation types that we will go through below. However, as ever it is important to look at the assignment guidance, as the word limits and section headings you will need to include are going to differ.

- **Primary research:** In this type of dissertation you carry out original research of your own, such as a survey or interviews (it would be very unusual for you to be able to do any clinical research for your dissertation, although it is not completely unheard of).
- **Literature review:** This sort of dissertation is a review of the existing literature on your topic.
- **Structured review:** This is sometimes called an evidence-based practice dissertation. A lot of dissertations in healthcare are a variant of a systematic review, using a structured question to do a literature search. They will often include a methodology chapter outlining how the literature search will be carried out.
- **Service improvement project:** A dissertation by another name with some added extras. This is all about identifying an area of improvement and then working through the steps to effectively either get to a point where it could be implemented or to implement it.

    Firstly we are going to have a look at the two types of reviews.

CHOOSING A TOPIC AND A TITLE

It sounds quite flippant to say the most important thing about your dissertation is the title, but everything does depend on it. Everything that you write in your dissertation should answer your question. You don't want to choose a topic that is too big, or you will never be able to answer it; or too narrow because there won't be enough research done on your topic for you to write a whole dissertation.

First make sure you find a subject you are interested in. Your dissertation will effectively take over your educational life until it is submitted, so start considering possible areas early in your course. Consider what you have seen during placements, as this would be a good starting point to identify an area of study. What really interested you?

Examples of dissertation topics:
- Specific management of a condition (e.g., prehospital stroke care, or prehospital end-of-life care).
- Investigation of a specific piece of equipment (e.g., the use of cervical collars in trauma, or gold-standard spinal care following blunt trauma).

TURNING YOUR TOPIC INTO A TITLE

Once you have got your topic you need to narrow this down into a more specific question. To do this, you need to get a feel for how big your topic is and how much there is out there.

You could do a 'quick and dirty' literature search, which involves typing your subject into Google Scholar and seeing what, if anything, comes up. For example, if we decided we were interested in paramedics cauterizing nosebleeds (epistaxis) prehospital, we might type in 'prehospital cauterization of epistaxis' and look through the hits. We get nothing that relates to prehospital care, so we would reconsider our subject. If we tried one of our areas of interest, 'prehospital end-of-life care by paramedics', there is quite a lot of research that is displayed, so it is worth carrying out a literature search. Just remember that a quick and dirty search is just for you—do not include it in your write-up. Try to consider as many search terms as possible. See Chapter 5 for more details. This should give you an idea of how big your topic area is. You want to find a topic for which some information is available—unless you are undertaking primary research, then getting very few hits is justification for researching the subject. Once you have done a bit of reading you will have more of an idea.

In healthcare we often use structured questions to form dissertation questions. Have a look at Chapter 2 to find out more.

DISSERTATION PROPOSALS

Often you will be asked to write a dissertation proposal as preparation for doing your main dissertation, often as part of a different module. If you are asked to do this in a different module, think ahead and don't waste your time doing a completely different subject: try to pick the subject you wish to undertake your dissertation on. Less work is always a plus.

This gives you the chance to consider how viable your dissertation idea is before you start to write it. It also gives your lecturers the chance to check that you are not going to try to do anything whacky. The good thing about doing a dissertation proposal is that you can get feedback on your dissertation idea before you start it. Sometimes your topic won't work, and you will need to modify it a bit to make it more suitable. You are more likely to be asked to do a dissertation proposal if you are doing primary research. If this is the case, then you are likely to need to complete an ethics form at the same time.

What your lecturers look for in a dissertation proposal:
- Whether you have chosen a relevant topic and title
- That the proposed research is something that you can realistically do
- That you have an appropriate methodology
- That what you are going to do is ethical
- That you have identified appropriate literature

STRUCTURING YOUR DISSERTATION

There are three main types of dissertation structures (Table 13.1). Your university might require something slightly different, but as you can see there is a lot of overlap.

Table 13.1 Dissertation Structures		
PRIMARY RESEARCH	**LITERATURE REVIEW**	**STRUCTURED REVIEW**
• Title page	• Title page	• Title page
• Abstract	• Abstract	• Abstract
• Table of contents	• Table of contents	• Table of contents
• Introduction	• Introduction	• Introduction
• Literature review	• Themed chapter	• Methodology
• Methodology	• Themed chapter	• Findings
• Findings	• Themed chapter	• Discussion
• Discussion	• Conclusion	• Conclusion
• Conclusion	• Bibliography	• Bibliography
• Bibliography	• Appendices	• Appendices
• Appendices		

Abstract

This is a one-paragraph summary of the whole of your dissertation. It comes before everything else in the dissertation, but it is good to write this last.

There are three main things you need to include:

- Your research question and the purpose of the research
- The methods you used
- Your findings and conclusion

Example (this is completely fictional and has not been researched in any way):

ABSTRACT

Research question: Should fast-response paramedics be allowed to sleep while on duty?

Purpose of research: There has been a longstanding debate between fast-response car drivers and management as to whether or not fast-response paramedics should be able to sleep on duty. The purpose of this review is to identify the evidence to weigh up the risks and benefits surrounding sleeping whilst on duty.

Methodology: A systematic review was undertaken using numerous academic databases. Multiple filters were applied to yield 37 research papers. Using a critiquing framework this was narrowed further to identify four relevant papers.

Findings: Four themes were identified within this review, these being: **the time available to sleep, the location of the fast-response vehicle**, and **the professionalism of the paramedic** and finally **the restorative nature of napping**.

Conclusion: The question is multifaceted. If the paramedic has over 20 minutes to nap, it can have a restorative effect and can help improve performance, especially during night shifts. Should the paramedic get less than 20 minutes of sleep, it will have the opposite effect. It was also deemed to look unprofessional and to reduce confidence in the paramedic should they be seen to be napping while on standby. Therefore the conclusion can be drawn that fast-response paramedics should not sleep on duty unless on an official timed meal break because the risks outweigh the benefits.

> Check with your module lecturer—often you should not include references in your abstract, but you do need to make sure.

INTRODUCTION

This should give a general background to your topic. It is helpful to think of the structure of the introduction as an upside-down triangle.

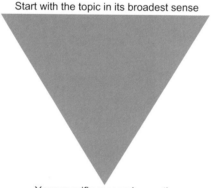

Start with the topic in its broadest sense

Your specific research question

John Swales (1980) identified that research paper introductions have a common structure which is also relevant to the introduction of your dissertation. He called this structure CARS, which stands for 'carving a research space'. An introduction has three stages (he calls them moves):

- **Establishing the territory:** This is where you tell us what your topic is and why it is important.
- **Identifying a niche:** Next you identify what aspect of the topic you are going to be researching. You should demonstrate that this is a gap in our knowledge (why else would you be researching it?).
- **Occupying the niche:** This is where you outline the purpose of your research. Tell us why it is important and give an overview of how you are going to go about it by outlining the structure of your dissertation.

It is important that the introduction is a good reflection of the rest of the dissertation. If you write your introduction early on, and your dissertation develops differently, you need to go back and edit so that it reflects this.

Some things you should include:

- What is your topic? Start with the general area.
- Give some facts and figures from professional sources.
- Provide definitions of any difficult terms. Try to use a definition from an expert in your field, rather than from a general dictionary.
- Offer your interpretation of the topic. Why is it important? What is the reason this topic needs writing about?
- Outline the main ideas or problems that stem from your topic. You must present these ideas in the exact order they will be dealt with in the main body of the dissertation.
- Sometimes your research question will come at the end of the introduction. It may be more appropriate to put it in your methodology.

INTRODUCTION EXTRACT

This example is just the starting three sentences; again **not** based on fact, with made up facts and figures!

> According to The National Office for Paramedics (2051) there are one million trauma calls per year that require rapid extraction from vehicles. Rapid extraction can be defined as removal of patients from the vehicle as quickly as possible owing to the severe nature of their injuries and the clinical investigations required (Professor 2050). In the United Kingdom alone there are 500 calls per year, a 4% rise in the last 6 months of 2052 (Nation Entrapment College 2053). This has led to 200 deaths in a 12-month period, a rise of 6% from the same period the previous year.

LITERATURE REVIEW

Sometimes your dissertation will have a separate literature review. Sometimes your dissertation itself will be a literature review, and therefore the literature review will be the findings chapter. To write your literature review, you need to have done a lot of reading.

The key thing about a literature review is it reviews the findings thematically, so we get a picture of what we already know about the topic and what we still need to find out. What it does not do is describe the articles one by one.

A lot of people would write something along the lines of the example in Box 13.1 (but possibly on a less frivolous topic).

However, this is not a good example of what to do. It is very descriptive and does not make any links between the studies. Sometimes this is described as a 'shopping list' approach, as it just lists one study after the other. What you need to do is to group and categorize the studies.

This example is thematic. It has grouped all research in the same area together. The idea is that you have a synthesis of findings and you can compare and contrast different research outcomes. Box 13.2 illustrates you should aim for.

Box 13.1 Literature Review 1

Teapot (2018) carried out a study which investigated digestive biscuits. She established that they are sold under a variety of different brand names, as well as being available in the chocolate variety. Of these varieties, she argues that the classic plain digestive biscuit is the most popular.

Crumb's study (2017) discovered an overwhelming preference for chocolate digestives. This quantitative study surveyed 525 people, 85% of whom preferred the chocolate variety. However, this group was divided, with 45% preferring dark chocolate digestives and 40% preferring the milk chocolate ones.

Tetley et al.'s qualitative study (2020) described the biscuit-eating experiences of 15 paramedics over a period of 6 months. They found that the paramedics preferred to have their biscuits with tea, with four participants saying that they were concerned that they were addicted to biscuits, with chocolate digestives being particularly moreish.

Box 13.2 Literature Review 2

Preference

The evidence suggests that there is a preference for chocolate digestives over the plain variety. Crumb's survey (2017) of 525 people found that 85% preferred chocolate digestives, with 40% favouring milk and 45% preferring dark chocolate. This is supported by Crunch's research (2013), in which 71% of the 100 people surveyed also preferred chocolate digestives. In contrast to this, Teapot (2018) argues that the classic plain digestive biscuit is the most popular; however, it is unclear what her evidence is for this claim.

Dependence

The second significant theme of the literature is that people became dependent upon digestive biscuits. Tetley et al.'s qualitative study (2020) investigated the biscuit-eating habits of 15 paramedics over a period of 6 months. Four of those in the study described developing a dependence on chocolate digestives. Although this is a very small-scale study, it does provide a detailed picture of how biscuit dependency develops over time. Crumb (2017) also found that 20% of those in her survey agreed with the statement 'I am worried about becoming dependent on digestive biscuits'.

Obviously, this sort of writing requires a lot more thought than the previous example because you need to make connections between ideas. You may need to include slightly more references in each section.

You should identify any areas that contradict each other (where there are two differing viewpoints) and identify any gaps in the literature. If there is not much information available about your subject, then there is a need to research it; this should be a justification for investigating your chosen research area.

METHODOLOGY

In your methodology you explain how you are going to answer your research question and why that is an appropriate method. Break your chapter into different subheadings to take readers through the process, step by step. The example here is for a systematic review. Think about your research. What is similar and different?

Overview of chapter
1. Methodology
   - Why you chose to do a systematic review
2. Research question
   - How you developed your question; for example, the PICO method
3. Methods
   - Search strategy (databases used)
   - Inclusion and exclusion criteria
   - Flow chart
4. Analysis
   - Identify themes
   - Critical appraisal tool (Polit & Beck)

It is helpful to think of your methodology as being like the recipe for a cake (Fig. 13.1): someone else should be able to read it and know exactly what you did for your research and replicate it if necessary.

FINDINGS

In this section, you will report your results in a systematic way. How you will do this depends on the type of research that you did. Unless you have combined the findings section with the discussion, you should not speculate on the meaning of the results here.

If you have done a literature review (or structured review)–based dissertation, the findings chapter should be structured rather like the example in the literature review section; you need to group the findings into themes. If you have done original research, you should report what you found. If you did quantitative research, this will involve presenting the data in graphs and tables with supporting commentary. If your research is qualitative, you should describe what you found, organized into different categories and themes. This should be supported by quotes from your data.

What to include:
- Start by outlining your approach to analysing and presenting the data. You should also outline how you have organized and structured the chapter.
- You can use the research questions as a way of structuring the chapter. It should be clear in the chapter how you have answered the research questions. Make sure you remind the reader of your research question in this chapter.
- Use clearly labelled graphs and charts to present any statistical data.

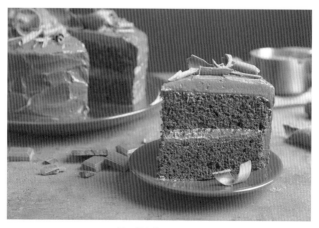

Fig. 13.1 Ummm cake.

- Note any inconsistencies in the findings. It is okay to identify inconsistencies in your findings, and in fact can add more value to your work.
- Include a short conclusion summarizing the findings and linking to the next chapter.
- If you have identified themes, then introduce them and link all the papers together.
- You should also discuss the quality of the information found (the validity of the research papers).

DISCUSSION

People often get confused about what goes in the discussion and what goes in the findings and the conclusion. Sometimes you will be asked to write a combined findings and discussion chapter. The difference is that in the findings chapter you report the results in a straightforward way, whereas in the discussion you comment in more detail about the findings. If there are any ambiguities or inconsistencies in the data, can you think of any reasons for this? How do your findings relate to practice? The findings section is for presenting the information, and the discussion is for looking at what all of it means and linking everything together.

This chapter should include:

- An introduction, where you give an overview of the chapter.
- A discussion of the significance of the findings. You could relate them back to the literature or to theory or professional practice.
- Discuss how generalizable the findings are. If you find you can support what you have written with other reputable sources, then you can introduce these too.

When you give explanations for your findings, you should use cautious language, for example: 'a possible reason for this could be' rather than 'this happened because'.

CONCLUSION

In your conclusion, you should aim to leave whoever is marking it with a good impression. Remind them what you have found out from doing your dissertation. How have you answered your research question? Remember, you want to sound confident in your conclusion:

- Start by restating your question(s).
- Next, summarize your findings. How have you added to what was already known (refer back to the literature)? Have you added anything new?
- What were the limitations of your research? Don't beat yourself up about them, all research has limitations, but it is important to acknowledge any factors that might have influenced the findings.
- Do you have any recommendations for further research? What do we still need to find out about?
- What are the implications of this research for professional practice (this is an area where you can show critical analysis and gain marks)?

Never introduce new information in any conclusion; work with what you have already identified.

DOING PRIMARY RESEARCH

Undertaking research is time-consuming and rather hard work. If the option is to undertake a literature review or undertake research, the choice is yours, but just make sure you engage with your supervisor early if you are considering primary research. Secondly, ensure that you understand what you are signing up to do and make sure you have the time to do it properly.

If you are doing any research of your own, the secret is to keep it simple. You obviously can't go off and do a big randomized controlled trial on your own, so focus your efforts on doing a small-scale study to the best of your ability. Here are some of the methods you could use if you are doing a research or service improvement project:

- **Surveys:** This is probably the easiest method to go with because you can reach a lot of people. You can hand out paper surveys or create online forms using software such as Survey Monkey or Microsoft Forms. Surveys can be used to collect different types of data. You can ask multiple choice questions, open questions or a mixture. It is important that you consider the wording carefully, so you don't ask leading questions. For example, 'can you tell me about your views on x?' is going to get a very different answer to 'can you tell me what is wrong with x?'.
- **Interviews:** If you are doing interviews, you need to think about what you are going to ask your participants and how you are going to word the questions. It is a good idea to practice your questions on a friend before you go off to ask them for real. It is also a good idea to record your interviews so you have an accurate account of what was said, but you will need to get the permission of the person you are interviewing to do so. You will need to transcribe the interview too, which does take a long time (at least 4 hours of transcription for every 1 hour of interview). There are some transcription software packages available; you will need to ask at your library.
- **Focus groups:** This is where you get a group of people together and ask them questions. You will need to ask fewer questions than you would in an interview of the same length, as there are more people talking. Some participants may feel more at ease in a group setting, and the group members will have the opportunity to share experiences

with each other. You will need to keep everyone on topic. The recordings of a focus group are really tricky to transcribe when it comes to writing it up.

When you write about the method you have chosen, you should explain why it is a suitable method for investigating your topic. You will need to provide references to support this. It is a good idea to get out a book on research methods to help you with this—there are lots.

If you are doing any kind of original research which involves people, you will need to think carefully about ethics. You didn't get to this point of your training (I hope) without realizing how important medical ethics is. You will need to fill out a university ethics form, and possibly even a NHS ethics form as well. Some of the things you will be asked to consider are:

- Informed consent
- Balance of power between researcher and participant (i.e., are they your patients?)
- Confidentiality
- How will you store the data?
- Is your method appropriate?
- General Data Protection Regulation (GPDR)
- Are there any safety issues?

You will need to produce informed consent forms for the participants and send them in with your ethics form for approval.

Once you have got all of these data, you are going to have to analyse them. You should consider what is the most appropriate form of analysis for your type of research and explain what you are going to do and why it is suitable.

Ethics is difficult, so if you do need ethics committee consent, then make sure you ask for help. At universities there are many people who have experience in this who would be more than willing to support you. Your supervisor can advise the best place to get help if he or she cannot help you himself or herself.

SERVICE IMPROVEMENT

In a service improvement project, you identify one aspect of the service that you would like to improve and make a plan of how you are going to improve it. Your project should be informed by both clinical evidence and service improvement tools. Just a point to note: if you read texts or the literature, service improvement is sometimes referred to as 'change'.

All universities will have slightly different requirements around service improvement projects, but some of the common aims are:

- For you to understand how evidence should be used to inform service changes and how you can go about this.
- To understand clinical governance, which is the system by which NHS organizations are accountable for continuously improving the quality of their services and safeguarding high standards of care Public Health England (2020).

WHAT TO INCLUDE

The problem with service improvement projects is that universities vary massively as to the expected content.

All require an introduction and a literature search, both of which are detailed above, but there are so many service improvement (or change) tools you can use that you need to check with your university as to their preferred methods.

CHANGE MODELS

There are different models that can be used to structure change within the NHS. The models presented here are those that will take you from the start to the finish of a project. They are important to know about (even just the name) because they might be something you can use in the future. Some of the most commonly used change models in healthcare are the NHS change model NHS (2018), Lewin's model and Kotters's model. These models will all have some helpful elements in them, but they describe the whole process from start to finish; whereas university service improvement projects usually stop once the issue has been identified and the service improvement recommendations have been made, predominantly because the ambulance service or hospitals can not afford to implement a whole cohort's ideas in a single year. That being said, it certainly does not mean that writing up a complete service improvement plan is a pointless exercise—you can present your ideas to the service, and maybe they will be so good that the service will work with you to implement it.

NHS Improving Quality has designed a simple guide to improving services (the reference is available at the end of the book) a bit of practice for you! The guide presents a five-step model that includes:

- **Preparation:** All the preparation you need to do. Consider it your introduction: aims, objectives, undertaking initial research—what is known, what is not and what exactly you are aiming to accomplish.
- **Launch:** Consider this your methodology. In effect, how are you going to undertake the project? How are you going to collect any data or information? In an actual project (where you plan to make the change) you would identify anyone you might work with and who will support you with the change.
- **Diagnosis:** This is all about looking at what is currently done and using data to actually demonstrate there is an issue. You need to do this with all projects of this nature: if it's not broke, don't fix it (remember this during your preparation phase—just because you don't like something doesn't mean it needs changing). You need to gather evidence to identify an actual improvement.

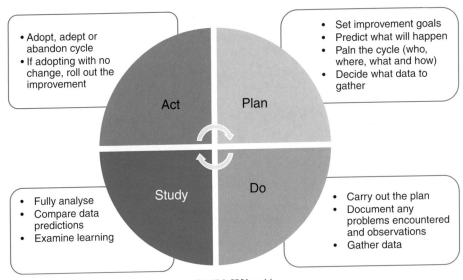

- Adopt, adept or abandon cycle
- If adopting with no change, roll out the improvement

Act

Plan

- Set improvement goals
- Predict what will happen
- Paln the cycle (who, where, what and how)
- Decide what data to gather

Study

Do

- Fully analyse
- Compare data predictions
- Examine learning

- Carry out the plan
- Document any problems encountered and observations
- Gather data

Fig. 13.2 PDSA model.

For some service improvements this where you would then make recommendations for change and conclude your work. For the service improvements that continue on to implementation, you carry on with the following two steps:

- **Implementation:** This is a testing phase, and a second model is brought in: the Plan Do Study Act model (Fig. 13.2).
- **Evaluation:** This is when you have a look at everything and then make recommendations for how to incorporate your service improvement into normal practice.

APPENDICES

In the course of writing any dissertation, you may have accrued lots of data. A brief synopsis within your work is good, but you will need to submit the rest in an appendix (meaning information at the end of your work, not the organ in your lower abdomen). Things like a gap analysis or a table of search terms for literature reviews can all be put in an appendix. Each item that you put in the appendix should be given a number or a letter that should be referred to in the main body of the report. The best part is, like the references, the appendix does not need to be included in your word count!

REFERENCES

As for all academic work, you need to include a comprehensive reference list. Instead of us waffling on about it again here, have a look at Chapter 4.

WRITING IT UP: THIS IS FOR ALL TYPES OF DISSERTATIONS

Where to start?

You have probably got the idea by now that you don't start writing your dissertation with the abstract and continue in page order. So where to begin? It is best to start with what you have got. In the very beginning, when you are still in the stage of turning your topic into a question, you will be reading a lot about the subject, and it is good to take some notes to keep track of what you have found out and what sense you can make of it.

Once you have worked out your question, you can create an outline of your whole dissertation. Break it down by chapter using headings and subheadings. You can use mind-mapping software or the headings and subheadings in Microsoft Word. Once you have created an outline, you can see which sections you are able to write. The methodology is often a good place to start. You can update your outline as the structure changes, but starting with at least a preliminary outline helps you keep track of the whole of your dissertation.

> Getting something (anything!) down on paper will help you feel organized and get you on your way, even if it is just the chapter headings.

It is a good idea to start writing early. This gives you the opportunity to get feedback on your work and check you are on the right line. Your supervisor can give you feedback on your writing (usually a small segment, you can't expect him or her to read the whole thing before you hand it in). Each university has their own guidance on how much time a supervisor has allocated to you. To make the most of this, you need to give your supervisor enough time to read and comment on your work and give yourself enough time to act on that feedback. There may also be a study skills service at your university where you can book a tutorial and get feedback on your writing.

Formatting is also important and can lose you marks if it is not done correctly. Many courses will give you a dissertation handbook that tells you how you need to format your dissertation. It might specify things like line spacing and fonts to use.

If you are using Microsoft Word, it is a good idea to use the headings and subheadings in Microsoft styles. This way you can create a table of contents which updates as you write.

HOW TO WRITE WHEN YOU DON'T WANT TO WRITE (KEEPING MOTIVATED)

Let's face it; it was not your life's dream to sit and write 10,000 words on resuscitation techniques. However interested in your topic you are, you are likely to have days when you hit the wall.

Bit of actual research for you now!

Research has found that the emotion people most associate with the writing process is 'frustration' (Brand 1990; Sword 2017). Alice Brand researched the emotions people feel around the writing process. She found that, while writing, positive emotions rose, and 'negative passive' emotions such as boredom and confusion decreased. Anxiety and frustration rose when people were actually writing but dropped off at the end. Relief and satisfaction peaked after a writing session. Interestingly, less skilled writers were more easily satisfied with their work than more skilled writers. If you are very critical about your own writing, this could be because you have high standards and are a good writer...not sure which category we fit into!

You might be the sort of person who always leaves writing assignments to the night before. This might be ok for an essay or a report, but this is not going to work for a dissertation. The best way to deal with this is to write little and often. Even if you only write a very small number of words each day, this builds up over a period of time (Fig. 13.3).

ONLINE WRITING MOTIVATION

There are lots of websites that can help motivate you to achieve your writing targets. The Pomodoro timer (www.online-stopwatch.com/pomodoro-timer/) is a timer you can use to time 25-minute bursts of writing. There are other websites which give you a reward (such as a picture of a cat) every time you reach a writing target, such as:

- Write or Die: http://writeordie.com/
- Written Kitten: https://writtenkitten.co/
- 750 words: https://750words.com/

Or there is always cake...if you do 500 words you get cake (or a nice apple if you are a health student). We always go with cake or chocolate; or even better, chocolate cake!

MANAGING YOUR WORKLOAD

Create a plan for completing your dissertation. Make a list of all of the tasks that you need to complete to finish your dissertation. You might identify extra things that you need to do once you are part way through the process but give it your best guess. Work backwards from your deadline. If you are the sort of person who likes graphs and spreadsheets you might want to make a Gantt chart (Fig. 13.4). This is a visual planning tool that breaks a project down into component tasks and creates a schedule for completing them.

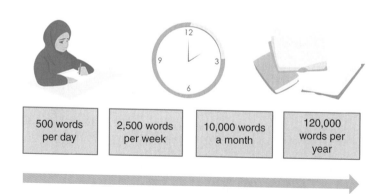

Fig. 13.3 Slow and steady equals good results.

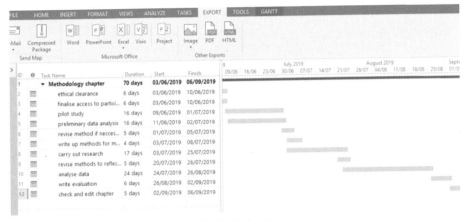

Fig. 13.4 Gantt chart.

Have a system for keeping track of all your references. If you are not already using reference management software, this might be a good time to start. See if your university subscribes to any—Write and Cite is a popular one. If that is not for you, then try keeping a separate Microsoft Word document or use the reference tool that comes with Microsoft Word.

> **Top Tip (Yep, of the Whole Book!):**
> Keep a backup copy of everything you do. Using online storage such as Google Docs is really useful because it will save as you go, so there is no reason to ever lose work again. You can also share it with your supervisor to stop lots of different copies going around.

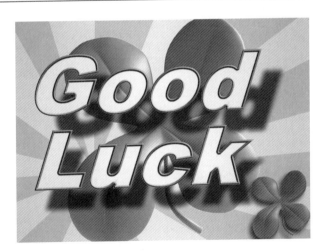

REFERENCES

Brand, A. (1990). Writing and feelings: checking our vital signs. *Rhetoric Review*, 8(2):290–308.

NHS. (2018). The change model guide [Online]. Available at: https://www.england.nhs.uk/wp-content/uploads/2018/04/change-model-guide-v5.pdf. Accessed on 31/07/2020.

NHS. (2020). Commission for quality and innovation. Available at: https://www.england.nhs.uk/nhs-standard-contract/cquin/. Accessed on 22/07/20.

Public Health England. (2020). Clinical governance. Available at: https://www.gov.uk/government/publications/newborn-hearing-screening-programme-nhsp-operational-guidance/4-clinical-governance. Accessed on 20/07/20.

Swales, J. M. (1990). *Genre analysis: English in academic and research settings*. New York: Cambridge University Press.

Sword, H. (2017). Air & Light & Time & Space, Harvard University Press, London.

KEY POINT SUMMARY AND HINTS AND TIPS

IN THIS CHAPTER:

- We give an overview of the key points of the book and provide some hints about studying at university.
- First, we look at reading and the different information sources you will use.
- Next we will discuss referencing.
- Then we will look at academic writing.
- Finally, we will present an overview of the different types of assessments.

If you only have time to read one chapter, read this one! This is an overview of the main ideas in the book.

INTRODUCTION TO STUDYING AT UNIVERSITY

You will learn at university through a combination of lectures, seminars and simulation, as well as your placements.

> Make sure you do the pre- and postlecture tasks because they often are designed to help with your final assessment.

At university you are responsible for your own study. No one is going to come and make you do it. However, there is a lot of support available to you. In your department you will have your subject lecturers and will be also given a personal tutor who you can go to. The university also makes support available from student welfare, disability support and the library (who often offer study skill support too). If you need help, ask for it.

READING AND FINDING INFORMATION

As a healthcare professional you will need to follow evidence-based practice. This means that you will have to read the evidence. You will need to provide a reference for everything that you have read.
You will be given a reading list with suggested things to read, but you will also have to learn how to find some for yourself. Textbooks are easier to read than some other sources, such as journal articles, so are a good starting point. You don't need to read everything on the reading list; you don't even need to read the whole book or article. Use the index in the back of the book to search for relevant information.

DOING A LIBRARY SEARCH

The first thing you need to do when you do a library search is to come up with some search terms. Think about what you want to find out and choose key words to describe your topic. Consider whether there any alternative words for your topic. For example, if you are researching paramedics and end-of-life care you might want to use the key words

'paramedics AND end-of-life care'. This might identify 3000 articles or none at all, so you could add other words to your search to increase or decrease the number of articles you retrieve. For example, you could put in 'paramedics OR ambulance AND end-of-life care OR palliative care'.

Remember that even if the research is of good quality, if it does not apply to you or the subject, then do not use it just for the sake of it.

Prioritize your reading and only read what you have to in order to answer the question. Always scan a text to make sure it's relevant before reading the whole thing; otherwise you will just get word blind, and nothing will make sense. Don't waste your time!

Keep track of everything that you read to save time later. Make sure you note down the full referencing details of any information you store; then it will be easier to compile your reference list at the end of your work. Do not just copy out what it says in the book. When you come back to your notes you need to be able to tell what are your ideas and words and what are the authors' to avoid accidentally committing plagiarism.

REFERENCING

Every time you claim something is a fact you will need to give a reference for it. In healthcare subjects, lecturers can be quite strict on referencing, so if in doubt it is better to put one in. There are different types of referencing styles. Harvard is the one that is most commonly used in healthcare subjects, so we have gone with that in this book, but your university will have its own guidance on this, so check with them. There is likely to be support available from your university library.

- Every time you claim something is a fact you need to include a reference.
- There are different styles of referencing, and you need to make sure you use the one that is accepted on your course.
- You can include evidence as a summary, paraphrase or direct quote.

There are two parts to referencing: a marker in the text and the full reference, which goes in the reference list at the end.

IN-TEXT CITATIONS

For example: 'According to Khan (2019)...'.

If the author's name is not part of the sentence, then you write your summary or paraphrase and then put the name and date just after. For example: 'Hip fractures are more common in people with osteoporosis (NHS 2020)'.

IN THE REFERENCE LIST

How you write the full reference depends on the type of source you have. This example is a book with just one author:

Author Surname, Initial(s). (Year). *Title*. Edition (if not first edition). Place of publication: Publisher.

For example:

Collen, A. (2017). *Decision making in paramedic practice*. Bridgwater: Class Publishing.

All the references should be listed in alphabetical order (by author's last name).

To put your reference list in order, you can use the A–Z sort function in Microsoft Word (found on the Home tab). Highlight the entire list and press the button. Alternatively, you can use reference management software to help you organize your reference list.

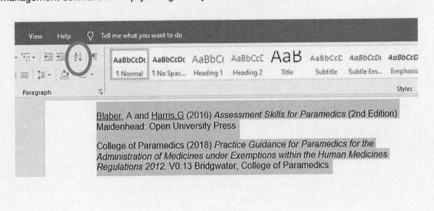

ACADEMIC WRITING

For all your university assignments you need to write in an academic style. There are a few features that make writing academic. These are:
- Formal style
- Evidence-based
- Cautious in tone
- Critical

FORMAL

Academic writing needs to be formal. This does not mean that you need to use fancy words, but you do need to:
- Avoid using colloquialisms. These are phrases that can be used in everyday language, such as 'at the end of the day' or 'I wasn't born yesterday'.
- Use the full version of words rather than the abbreviated version. For example: 'do not' rather than 'don't', 'defibrillator' rather than 'defib', 'technology' rather than 'tech'…you get the drift (this is a colloquialism, by the way).
- Avoid using emotive language. Sometimes if you are discussing something you are passionate about it, this can be difficult, but avoiding words such as 'tragically', 'dreadful' or 'horrifically' can actually mean your work is taken more seriously.

EVIDENCE BASED

Make sure any key information you are putting in your assignment or paper is supported by evidence; otherwise your work will not be taken seriously, and you will get a low grade or be unable to publish your paper.

Remember that, in general, academic writing uses the third person. However, there are exceptions to this; for example, in reflective writing it is usual to write in the first person.

CRITICAL WRITING

Critical writing means that you question assumptions and don't take things at face value. It doesn't mean that you need to be negative. Your work should have an argument (an answer to the question) and be structured in a logical way, with a clear introduction and conclusion.

One way to structure your work is by using the Point, Evidence, Explanation, Link (PEEL) paragraph structure. All paragraphs should have one main point which you develop throughout.

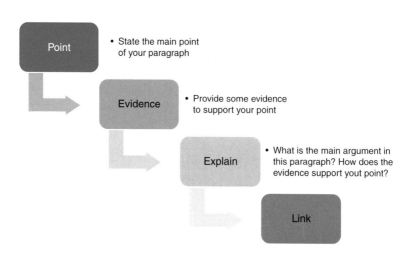

Point
- State the main point of your paragraph

Evidence
- Provide some evidence to support your point

Explain
- What is the main argument in this paragraph? How does the evidence support yout point?

Link

TYPES OF ASSESSMENT

Throughout your time at university, you will have to do a variety of different types of assignments. Every assignment you do should come with 'learning outcomes' (which, unsurprisingly, are what you are meant to learn) and assessment criteria (how it will be marked). These guidelines give you an insight into what the lecturers will be looking for. Make sure that you read them carefully and include everything that you need to include.

ESSAYS

Box 14.1 illustrates essay structure.

Box 14.1 Essay Structure

Introduction (around 10% of the word count)
- What is the **context**? Provide some background information about the topic
- Define **key terms**
- What is **this essay** about (how have you interpreted the question, and what will you focus on)? If you have been given a choice of what to write about, make it clear what you have chosen
- **Structure**. Introduce the main ideas in the order that you will cover them

Main Body (around 85% of the word count)
- Use a chain of paragraphs to explore and develop your ideas/argument
- You will probably have four or five main topics or themes. These can:
  - Be given to you in an assignment brief
  - Emerge from your reading or thinking (consider your mind map)
- Each topic or theme is explored in one or more paragraphs
- Consider the breakdown of the word count. For example, if each paragraph is 100–200 words, then each theme could be explored in 500 words, three paragraphs, etc.
- You can use the Point, Evidence, Explanation, Link approach to structure your paragraphs

Conclusion (around 5% of the word count)
- Do not introduce any new material here (if it is important, it needs to be included in the main body of the essay)
- Summarize your main argument. **How have you answered the question?**
- Why are your conclusions important or **significant**? Are there any wider implications?

EXAMS

There are three main types of exams you might have to take: traditional written exams, objective structured clinical examinations (OSCEs) and viva voce exams. First work out what you are being asked to include. Don't just waffle because it will only take up time.

Start by working out what you need to revise.

Before the exams:
- Find out:
  - When and where the exam will take place
  - The length of the exam
  - The number of questions
  - The time allowed for the exam
- Practice doing the exam to time, as this can help develop your writing speed
- Check key points such as parking and travel time
- Eat before going in
- And yes, use the loo; there is nothing worse than needing to go midexam (who can beat a nervous wee?)

OBJECTIVE STRUCTURED CLINICAL EXAMINATION

An OSCE is a practical exam where you will have to demonstrate clinical skills. You will be given a scenario that you will have to react to as if you are in practice. You will be marked for this, and there are some situations called 'critical fails' where, if you make a big mistake, you will fail the whole exam. A viva voce is a spoken exam (Box 14.2).

Box 14.2 Hints and Tips

Hints and tips for objective structured clinical examinations and viva voce examinations:
- Find out what is being tested and make sure you revise the correct subject.
- Use the time you have been given—try not to rush things. If you have time left over to recap exactly what you have done, you might remember something you have missed out.
- Dress professionally, either in a neat and tidy uniform or smart but practical clothing. Tie long hair up, and for the practical lesson make sure you are bare below the elbow (NHS guidance).
- Listen to the question or read any information sheets carefully—make sure you know what is being asked of you.

Do not just learn everything by rote (do not just learn your lines). If you actually understand what you are saying, then there is less of a chance of freezing in the middle of your OSCE.

Remember that you can often forget one or two areas (that are not critical fails) and still get enough points to pass the assessment. So, if you remember something you forgot to say when you leave, try not to panic.

Top Tip (Yep, of the Whole Book!)

Keep a backup copy of everything you do. Using online storage such as Google Docs is really useful, as it will save as you go, so there is no reason to ever lose work again. You can also share it with your supervisor to stop lots of different copies going around.

STUDY SKILLS FOR PARAMEDICS AND OTHER HEALTH CARE PROFESSIONALS

FULL REFERENCE LIST

Agarwal, R., & Baid, R. (2016). Asterixis. *Journal of Postgraduate Medicine, 62*(2), 115–117.

Alberti, R. E., & Emmons, M. L. (2017). *Your perfect right: Assertiveness and equality in your life and relationships.* (10th ed.). Oakland: New Harbinger Publications, Inc.

Benger, J. R., Kirby, K., & Black, S., et al. (2018). Effect of a strategy of a supraglottic airway device vs tracheal intubation during out-of-hospital cardiac arrest on functional outcome: The AIRWAYS-2 randomized clinical trial. *The Journal of the American Medical Association, 320*(8), 779–791.

Blaber, A., & Harris, G. (2016). *Assessment skills for paramedics.* (2nd ed.). Maidenhead: Open University Press.

Brand, A. (1990). Writing and feelings: Checking our vital signs. *Rhetoric Review, 8*(2), 290–308.

Centre for Reviews and Dissemination. (2008). *Systematic reviews: CRD's guidance for undertaking reviews in healthcare.* York: University of York. Available at: https://www.york.ac.uk/media/crd/Systematic_Reviews.pdf. Accessed on 14/06/2020.

Coats, T.J., Fragoso-Iñiguez, M., & Roberts, I. (2019). Implementation of tranexamic acid for bleeding trauma patients: A longitudinal and cross-sectional study. *Emergency Medicine Journal, 36*, 78–81.

College of Paramedics. (2018). *Practice guidance for paramedics for the administration of medicines under exemptions within the Human Medicines Regulations 2012.* (Vol 13). Bridgwater: College of Paramedics.

Collen, A. (2017). *Decision making in paramedic practice.* Bridgwater: Class Publishing.

Cooke, A., Smith, D., & Booth, A. (2012). Beyond PICO: The SPIDER tool for qualitative evidence synthesis. *Qualitative Health Research, 22*(10),1435–1443.

Cox, N. (2016). Cardiovascular system. In: T. A. Roper (Ed.), *Clinical skills,* (2nd ed, pp. 28–83). Oxford: Oxford University Press.

Department for Education. (2018). *Working together to safeguard children: A guide to inter-agency working to safeguard and promote the welfare of children [Online].* London: Department for Education. Available at: https://assets.publishing. service.gov.uk/government/uploads/system/uploads/attachment_data/file/722305/Working_Together_to_Safeguard_ Children_-_Guide.pdf.

Department of Health. (2015). *Mental Health Act 1983: Code of practice [Online].* London: The Stationery Office. Available at: https://assets.publishing.service.gov.uk/government/uploads/system/uploads/attachment_data/file/435512/MHA_ Code_of_Practice.PDF. Accessed on 17/04/2020.

Eaton. (2019). *Law and ethics for paramedics.* Bridgwater: Class Publishing.

Ennis, P. (2019). A pilot of the Paramedic Advanced Resuscitation of Children (PARC) course. *Journal of Paramedic Practice, 11*(11).

Gibbs, G. (1988). *Learning by doing: A guide to teaching and learning methods.* Oxford Further Educational Unit: Oxford Polytechnic.

Glover, J., Izzo, D., Odato, K., et al. (2006). *EBM pyramid.* Dartmouth University/Yale University.

Glover, T. E., Sumpter, J. E., Ercole, A., et al. (2019). Pulmonary embolism following complex trauma: UK MTC observational study. *Emergency Medicine Journal, 36*(10), 608–612.

Greenhalgh, T. (2019). *How to read a paper: The basics of evidence based medicine,* (6th ed.). London: Wiley Blackwell.

HCPC. (2016). *Standards of conduct, performance and ethics.* Available at: https://www.hcpc-uk.org/standards/standards-of-conduct-performance-and-ethics/. Accessed on 12/05/2020.

HESA. (2020). *Figure 4 - HE student enrolments by personal characteristics 2014/15 to 2018/19.* Available at: https://www. hesa.ac.uk/data-and-analysis/sb252/figure-4. Accessed on 31/07/2020.

Hilsdon, J. (2010). *Critical thinking.* Available at: https://www.plymouth.ac.uk/uploads/production/document/path/1/1710/ Critical_Thinking.pdf. Accessed on 31/07/2020.

Howick, J., Chalmers, I., Glasziou, P., et al. (2021). *Explanation of the 2011 Oxford Centre for Evidence-Based Medicine (OCEBM) Levels of Evidence (Background Document).* Oxford Centre for Evidence-Based Medicine. Available at: https:// www.cebm.ox.ac.uk/resources/levels-of-evidence/ocebm-levels-of-evidence.

Howick, J., Chalmers, I., Glasziou, P., et al. (2021). *The 2011 Oxford CEBM Evidence Levels of Evidence (Introductory Document).* Oxford Centre for Evidence-Based Medicine. Available at: https://www.cebm.ox.ac.uk/resources/levels-of-evidence/ocebm-levels-of-evidence.

Izawa, J., et al. (2019). Pre-hospital advanced airway management for adults with out-of-hospital cardiac arrest: Nationwide cohort study. *British Medical Journal, 364*, l430.

Middlebrook, R. D. (1994). *Using scrolls [Online]*. Available at: http://www.textmapping.org/using.html. Accessed on 31/07/2020.

Moher D., Liberati A., Tetzlaff J., et al. (2009). Preferred reporting items for systematic reviews and meta-analyses: The PRISMA statement. *PLoS Medicine, 6*(7), e1000097.

NHS. (2016). *Major trauma centres in England [Online]*. Available at: https://www.nhs.uk/NHSEngland/AboutNHSservices/Emergencyandurgentcareservices/Documents/2016/MTS-map.pdf. Accessed on 14/06/2020.

NHS. (2018). *Complications, severe head injury*. Available at: https://www.nhs.uk/conditions/severe-head-injury/complications/. Accessed on 15/05/2020.

NHS. (2018). *The change model guide [Online]*. Available at: https://www.england.nhs.uk/wp-content/uploads/2018/04/change-model-guide-v5.pdf. Accessed on 31/07/2020.

NHS. (2019). *Assessing capacity*. Available at: https://www.nhs.uk/conditions/consent-to-treatment/capacity/. Accessed on 25/03/2020.

NHS. (2020). *Commissioning for quality and innovation*. Available at: https://www.england.nhs.uk/nhs-standard-contract/cquin/. Accessed on 22/07/2020.

NICE. (2012). *Significant haemorrhage following trauma: Tranexamic acid [Online]*. Available at: https://www.nice.org.uk/advice/esuom1/chapter/key-points-from-the-evidence. Accessed on 4/06/2020.

NICE. (2014). *Head injury; quality standards*. Available at: https://www.nice.org.uk/guidance/qs74/chapter/quality-statement-2-ct-head-scans-for-people-taking-anticoagulants. Accessed on 15/05/2020.

NICE. (2016). *Fractures (non-complex): Assessment and management [Online]*. Available at: https://www.nice.org.uk/guidance/NG38/chapter/Recommendations#acute-stage-assessment-and-diagnostic-imaging. Accessed on 31/07/2020.

OCEBM Levels of Evidence Working Group. (2011). The Oxford levels of evidence 2. *PLoS Medicine, 6*(7), e1000097. Available at: https://www.cebm.net/index.aspx?o=5653. Accessed on 31/07/2020.

Public Health England. (2020). *Clinical governance*. Available at: https://www.gov.uk/government/publications/newborn-hearing-screening-programme-nhsp-operational-guidance/4-clinical-governance. Accessed on 20/07/2020.

SEEC. (2016). *Credit level descriptors for higher education – 2016 [Online]*. Available at: https://seec.org.uk/wp-content/uploads/2016/07/SEEC-descriptors-2016.pdf. Accessed on 11/06/2020.

Swales, J. M. (1990). *Genre analysis: English in academic and research settings*. New York: Cambridge University Press.

Sword, H. (2017). Air & Light & Time & Space, Harvard University Press, London.

University of Manchester. (2020). *Academic phrasebank [Online]*. Available at: http://www.phrasebank.manchester.ac.uk/. Accessed on 20/04/2020.

WHO. (2018). *Diabetes key facts*. Available at: https://www.who.int/news-room/fact-sheets/detail/diabetes. Accessed on 12/05/2020.

Willis, S. (2010). Becoming a reflective practitioner: Frameworks for the prehospital professional. *Journal of Paramedic Practice, 2*(5), 212–216.

Zhang, Z. J., Yu, X. J., Fu, T., et al. (2020). Novel coronavirus infection in newborn babies under 28 days in China. *European Respiratory Journal, 55*(6).

INDEX

Note: Page numbers followed by *f* indicate figures, *t* indicate tables, and *b* indicate boxes.